BRAIN FITNESS REVOLUTION

ENHANCE MEMORY, SHARPEN FOCUS, AND BOOST PRODUCTIVITY WITH PROVEN STRATEGIES

MILES STERLING

CONTENTS

Introduction — 7

1. **UNDERSTANDING MEMORY AND ITS CHALLENGES** — 11
   1.1 The Science of Memory: How We Remember — 11
   1.2 Common Memory Challenges and Misconceptions — 13
   1.3 The Impact of Stress on Memory Retention — 15
   1.4 Age-Related Memory Decline: Facts and Myths — 17
   1.5 Personalizing Your Memory Improvement — 19

2. **LAYING THE FOUNDATION FOR COGNITIVE ENHANCEMENT** — 23
   2.1 The Role of Nutrition in Memory Improvement — 26
   2.2 Mindfulness as a Tool for Better Focus — 28
   2.3 Setting Achievable Memory Improvement Goals — 31

3. **PROVEN MEMORY ENHANCEMENT TECHNIQUES** — 35
   3.1 Mnemonics: Crafting Effective Memory Aids — 37
   3.2 Chunking Information for Easier Recall — 39
   3.3 The Power of Repetition and Spacing Effect — 41
   3.4 Leveraging Storytelling to Enhance Memory — 43

4. **PRACTICAL DAILY EXERCISES FOR MEMORY BOOST** — 47
   4.1 Lunchtime Neurobics: Break Routine with Cognitive Workouts — 49
   4.2 Evening Reflection: Consolidating Daily Learning — 51
   4.3 Weekend Memory Challenges: Fun Exercises for Families — 53
   4.4 Tracking Progress: How to Measure Your Memory Improvement — 55

5. **ADAPTING EXERCISES TO YOUR COGNITIVE LEVEL** — 59
   5.1 Intermediate Challenges: Building on Basics — 61
   5.2 Advanced Techniques: Pushing Cognitive Limits — 63

5.3 Customizing Exercises for Personal Preferences ... 65
5.4 Overcoming Plateaus in Memory Improvement ... 67

6. USING TECHNOLOGY TO AID MEMORY IMPROVEMENT ... 73
   6.1 Virtual Reality: Immersive Memory Training ... 75
   6.2 Gamifying Memory Exercises for Motivation ... 77
   6.3 Digital Tools for Tracking Memory Progress ... 79
   6.4 Integrating Technology with Traditional Techniques ... 81

7. ADDRESSING COMMON MEMORY IMPROVEMENT BARRIERS ... 85
   7.1 Managing Time: Incorporating Exercises into Busy Schedules ... 87
   7.2 Dealing with Discouragement: How to Stay Motivated ... 89
   7.3 Finding Support: Building a Memory Improvement Community ... 91
   7.4 Communicating Your Memory Needs to Family and Friends ... 93

8. HOLISTIC APPROACHES TO COGNITIVE HEALTH ... 97
   8.1 The Connection Between Physical Health and Memory ... 97
   8.2 Stress Management Techniques for Better Memory ... 99
   8.3 Sleep and Its Role in Memory Consolidation ... 101
   8.4 The Impact of Social Interaction on Cognitive Function ... 103
   8.5 Creating a Balanced Lifestyle for Optimal Memory Health ... 105

9. REAL-LIFE SUCCESS STORIES AND TESTIMONIALS ... 109
   9.1 Lessons Learned: What Worked for Others ... 112
   9.2 Overcoming Setbacks: Stories of Persistence ... 113
   9.3 The Power of Community in Memory Improvement ... 115
   9.4 Testimonials: Voices of Those Who Remember ... 118

10. SUSTAINING MEMORY IMPROVEMENT FOR LIFE	121
10.1 Future-Proofing Your Memory: Trends and Innovations	124
10.2 Celebrating Your Memory Journey: Milestones and Achievements	126
Conclusion	129
References	133

INTRODUCTION

Memory is more important than ever in a world where information bombards us every second. Consider this: by age 40, many people notice a decline in their ability to recall names or remember where they left their keys. It's a startling reality. We rely on our memory for so much—from daily tasks to cherished moments. Yet, memory loss isn't just an inevitable part of aging. It's a challenge we can tackle.

Memory was once my superpower. I could remember faces, names, and even phone numbers with ease. Day planners were for others, not for someone like me. But as the years went by, I found myself reaching for that planner more and more. When I retired, I relied on an app to remind me of daily tasks, medications, and appointments. It was a gradual shift, a silent thief taking bits of my memory.

This shift motivated me to dig deeper. I sought every trick, game, and method that promised a sharper memory. But time and again, I found myself disappointed. Nothing worked. So, I turned to research. I became fascinated by why memory declines and how we might reclaim it. This journey of discovery has led to this guide, a tool to help you enhance or preserve your memory.

The purpose of this book is simple. I want to offer you easy, practical exercises to improve your memory. These techniques can fit seamlessly into your daily routine. You don't need to carve out hours from your busy day. Instead, these exercises are designed to be quick and effective, providing accurate results without overwhelming your schedule.

Cognitive improvement is more than just remembering where you parked your car. It's about sharpening your focus, increasing productivity, and enhancing your quality of life. Whether dealing with memory challenges or looking to stay sharp, cognitive improvement is the key to unlocking a brighter future.

Imagine focusing better at work, breezing through tasks, and enjoying a more vibrant social life. These are just a few of the benefits memory enhancement can offer. The exercises in this book will boost your memory and improve your overall cognitive health. The positive outcomes extend beyond memory, touching every aspect of your life.

In the chapters ahead, we'll start by understanding memory itself—what it is, how it works, and why it sometimes fails us. We'll dive into practical exercises and strategies to improve long-term memory. Each chapter builds on the last, guiding you through a transformation journey.

You might have concerns. You may have tried other methods before and found them lacking. Or you may need to be more skeptical about whether such exercises can make a difference. Rest assured, this book is grounded in evidence-based approaches. The exercises here are tested and proven, designed to be practical and effective.

As you turn these pages, keep an open mind and embrace the journey ahead. The potential for significant improvement is accurate, and personal growth is within your reach. We'll explore strategies to transform how you think, remember, and live together.

Let this book be your guide. Let's embark on this journey to sharpen our memory, enhance our focus, and boost our productivity. Your path to cognitive improvement begins here. The changes you seek are possible, and the journey to a better memory starts now.

CHAPTER ONE
UNDERSTANDING MEMORY AND ITS CHALLENGES

Have you ever walked into a room only to forget why you went there in the first place? You're not alone. Many of us experience such moments where the mind seems to betray us. These instances, though frustrating, are part of the complex world of memory. This chapter will guide you through the intricate processes of how memory works and why it sometimes falters. Understanding these mechanisms is the first step in reclaiming control over your memory. By diving into the science behind it, you will uncover the fascinating roles of different brain parts and how they contribute to the tapestry of our memories.

1.1 THE SCIENCE OF MEMORY: HOW WE REMEMBER

Memory is a marvel of the mind, orchestrated by processes that transform fleeting moments into lasting impressions. At the heart of this marvel are three key stages: encoding, storage, and retrieval. Encoding is the initial phase where information is translated into a form the brain can understand. This stage is crucial as it determines how well you can recall information later. Think of it as the brain's way of taking notes on daily experiences. Once encoded, information moves to storage, which is preserved over time. This storage can be short-term or long-term. Short-term memory holds information temporarily, like remembering a phone number long enough to dial it. In contrast, long-term memory stores knowledge more permanently, allowing you to recall childhood memories or the lyrics of your favorite song. Retrieval is the final step, enabling you to access stored information when needed, whether recalling what you had for breakfast or the name of a distant cousin.

Central to these processes are specific brain structures. The hippocampus, nestled within the temporal lobe, plays a pivotal role in converting short-term memories into long-term ones. This region acts as a memory librarian, cataloging experiences for future reference. Damage to the hippocampus, such as from injury or disease, can severely impact your ability to form new memories, underscoring its importance. Working alongside the hippocampus is the amygdala, a small almond-shaped structure responsible for emotional memories. It ensures that emotional experiences, such as the joy of a wedding day or the fear of a near-accident, are vividly etched in your mind. The interplay between the hippocampus and amygdala is crucial, as it helps create rich, emotional tapestries of your past.

Neuroplasticity is another fascinating aspect of memory. This concept refers to the brain's incredible ability to reorganize by forming new neural connections throughout life. It's why you can learn new skills or recover from brain injuries. For instance, learning to play a musical instrument or mastering a new language can enhance neuroplasticity, reinforcing your brain's capacity to adapt and thrive. This adaptability has profound implications for memory exercises, offering hope that consistent practice can lead to meaningful improvements, regardless of age or previous memory challenges.

Memory isn't a singular entity but a collection of types, each serving different functions. Procedural memory, for example, is responsible for skills and tasks like riding a bike or typing on a keyboard. You can perform these actions without consciously thinking about each step. On the other hand, declarative memory concerns facts and information, helping you recall historical dates or the capital of a country. Within declarative memory, episodic memory allows you to remember personal experiences, like your last vacation. In contrast, semantic memory involves general knowledge, such as understanding the concept of gravity without recalling when or where you learned it. Each type of memory contributes to the rich tapestry of your cognitive life, allowing you to navigate the world with a blend of learned skills and acquired knowledge.

1.2 COMMON MEMORY CHALLENGES AND MISCONCEPTIONS

Memory challenges manifest in various forms, from forgetting why you entered a room to more persistent difficulties like recalling recent conversations or misplacing everyday items. These lapses, though common, can be distressing, leading many to question their cognitive health. Concentration and focus are also frequent hurdles. In our fast-paced world, distractions abound, making it harder to focus on tasks. Whether it's the constant ping of notifications or the multitasking culture many of us are entrenched in, staying focused has become a modern-day challenge. These issues can lead to cognitive overload, where the mind feels cluttered and unable to process information efficiently.

Amidst these concerns, several misconceptions about memory persist. One prevalent belief is that memory loss is an unavoidable part of aging. While it's true that specific cognitive changes occur as we grow older, it doesn't mean memory decline is inevitable or irreversible. Many people also mistakenly think they can't improve it once memory slips. This myth can deter individuals from seeking solutions that could significantly enhance their memory capabilities. Another misunderstanding is that memory aids, like mnemonics or reminders, are unnecessary or even a sign of weakness. On the contrary, these tools can be incredibly effective in supporting memory retention and should be embraced as helpful strategies rather than avoided.

The impact of lifestyle choices on memory is profound. Nutrition plays a pivotal role in cognitive function. Diets lacking essential nutrients can impair brain health, leading to difficulties in memory retention. A balanced diet of fruits, vegetables, lean proteins, and healthy fats supports cognitive well-being. Sleep is another crucial factor. Sleep deprivation disrupts the brain's ability to consolidate memories, making individuals foggy and forgetful. Ensuring adequate sleep rest allows the brain to process and store information effectively. Stress, too, can wreak havoc on memory. Chronic stress bombards the brain with stress hormones, which can impair memory recall and lead to cognitive decline.

Technology, with its myriad benefits, also poses challenges. Many of us rely on digital tools to keep track of appointments, tasks, and even birthdays. While these aids are convenient, over-reliance can weaken our memory muscles. When we no longer need to remember because our devices do it for us, our brain's ability to recall naturally diminishes. Moreover, the constant barrage of information from screens can lead to cognitive overload, making it difficult to focus and retain essential details. The brain struggles to process the influx, leading to scattered thinking and reduced memory retention.

Interactive Element: Reflection Section

Take a moment to reflect on your daily habits. Consider how often you rely on technology for reminders. Jot down instances where you could challenge your memory instead, like recalling a friend's phone number or the ingredients for a recipe. This simple exercise can help identify areas where you can naturally strengthen your memory.

In addressing these challenges and misconceptions, it's crucial to recognize the potential for improvement. Memory isn't a static trait; it's a dynamic ability that can be nurtured and enhanced. By understanding the factors that influence memory, from lifestyle choices to technological reliance, we can take proactive steps to bolster our cognitive health. This book aims to provide the tools and knowledge to navigate these challenges, empowering you to reclaim and strengthen your memory.

1.3 THE IMPACT OF STRESS ON MEMORY RETENTION

Stress, an inevitable part of life, profoundly influences our minds, particularly memory. At the heart of this impact is cortisol, a stress hormone that surges through our system during high-pressure moments. This hormone plays a dual role, sometimes enhancing memory but often impairing it. The hippocampus, a critical brain region for memory, is susceptible to cortisol's effects. When stress levels rise, cortisol floods the hippocampus, disrupting its ability to process and store memories effectively. Over time, high cortisol levels can even alter the structure of the hippocampus, leading to memory lapses that range from misplacing keys to forgetting essential conversations. In chronic stress scenarios—think of a high-pressure job with endless demands or long-term caregiving—this persistent cortisol presence can degrade memory over the long haul, making it harder to recall even significant life events.

Yet, not all stress is detrimental. Short bursts, like the adrenaline rush before a presentation, can sharpen our focus and enhance memory recall. This acute stress temporarily boosts cognitive function, allowing us to remember details clearly. It's a survival mechanism, fine-tuned by evolution to help us respond to immediate threats. However, when stress becomes a constant companion, the benefits quickly diminish. Under relentless stress, the brain enters a state of constant alert, which strains its resources and hampers memory retention. Chronic stress can seep into every corner of life, from workplace pressures to personal challenges, eroding cognitive function over time.

Effective stress management techniques are vital to counteract stress's grip on memory. Mindfulness practices, which focus on staying present, offer a way to reduce stress's hold on the brain. These techniques encourage a calm, focused mind through simple exercises like deep breathing and meditation. Regular physical exercise also plays a crucial role. Walking, yoga, or cycling improve overall health and help regulate cortisol levels, thus protecting memory function. Engaging in these activities releases endorphins, which improve mood and reduce stress, creating a more favorable environment for memory retention.

Relentless stress can lead to a vicious cycle, where memory lapses cause more stress, further impacting memory. Relaxation techniques have become invaluable in breaking this cycle. Simple practices like progressive muscle relaxation or calming music can soothe the mind and reduce cortisol levels. These methods help create a buffer against stress, allowing the hippocampus to recover and function optimally. By incorporating these relaxation practices into daily life, you can nurture a healthier brain environment that supports robust memory function even in the face of life's pressures.

Interactive Element: Stress Management Checklist

Identify three daily stressors. For each, list one mindfulness practice, one physical activity, and one relaxation technique you can use to manage the stress. This personalized checklist can help you proactively address stress, supporting better memory retention.

Understanding the nuanced relationship between stress and memory empowers you to take control. By recognizing the signs of stress and implementing strategies to manage it, you can safeguard your memory. This proactive approach not only improves cognitive health but also enhances overall well-being. Building resilience against stress's effects requires consistent effort, but the rewards—a clearer mind, improved memory, and a more balanced life—are well worth it.

1.4 AGE-RELATED MEMORY DECLINE: FACTS AND MYTHS

As the years add up, it's natural to notice changes in remembering things. However, only some forgetful moments are signs of trouble. Understanding what changes are typical can bring clarity and peace of mind. For instance, it's normal to occasionally forget where you put your glasses or why you walked into a room. These instances are often due to distractions or multitasking. However, when memory lapses interfere with daily life, such as forgetting how to perform routine activities or struggling to follow conversations, they may indicate a more serious issue that warrants attention. Recognizing these differences can help you determine when to seek professional advice.

A common myth suggests that aging automatically leads to significant memory loss. This belief can be discouraging, painting a grim picture of the future. Yet research provides a more hopeful narrative. While the brain changes with age, many older adults maintain robust cognitive abilities well into their later years. Studies have shown that engaging in mental activities—like reading, puzzles, or learning new skills—can preserve memory functions. Moreover, seniors who remain socially active often display better memory retention. The brain thrives on stimulation and novelty, debunking the myth that decline is unavoidable.

Recent research continues to shed light on memory preservation among older adults. Evidence suggests that those who keep their minds active through hobbies, education, and social engagement tend to fare better cognitively. Activities that challenge the brain, like playing musical instruments or learning a new language, have been linked to improved memory and delayed cognitive decline. This research underscores the importance of staying mentally active to maintain mental health. It also highlights the brain's adaptability, even as it ages, reinforcing that it's never too late to adopt new habits or hobbies that can bolster cognitive resilience.

Proactive strategies can be immensely beneficial to combat age-related memory decline. Cognitive exercises tailored for seniors, such as memory games, word puzzles, and brain-training apps, offer stimulating ways to keep the mind sharp. These activities can enhance memory by encouraging the brain to form new connections and strengthen existing ones. Social engagement also plays a crucial role. Regular interaction with family, friends, or community groups can provide mental stimulation and emotional support, contributing to better memory health. Participating in clubs, volunteering, or maintaining a regular social calendar can give your brain the necessary workout.

It's essential to approach memory changes with a balanced perspective, recognizing that while some decline is natural, it isn't inevitable or irreversible. By staying informed and adopting proactive measures, you can navigate the changes that come with aging more confidently. Remember, your brain remains a dynamic organ capable of growth and adaptation, even as you age.

1.5 PERSONALIZING YOUR MEMORY IMPROVEMENT

The first step is understanding where you currently stand before enhancing your memory. Assessing your memory needs involves closely examining your daily interactions and experiences. Consider when you struggle to recall names, details, or tasks. Are there specific times of the day when your memory seems sharper or more sluggish? These reflections will help identify areas needing attention. Simple self-assessment techniques can paint a clearer picture, such as jotting down moments of forgetfulness or areas where you excel. This informal inventory can reveal patterns and guide you in deciding which exercises might benefit you most.

Once you've gained insight into your memory strengths and weaknesses, setting personal goals becomes the next vital step. This process is similar to setting other life goals, requiring thoughtfulness and realism. Start by deciding what you want to improve. You may wish to recall names more efficiently or remember daily tasks without a list by setting specific yet achievable goals to motivate you and provide direction. Begin with small, attainable objectives and gradually increase the complexity as you progress. By aligning your memory goals with daily life, you create a personalized roadmap that makes success more achievable.

Tailoring memory exercises to fit your lifestyle is crucial for sustained improvement. Some people have different schedules or preferences, so it's essential to customize your approach. If you're a morning person, incorporating memory exercises into your morning routine might be ideal. For others, evening might be a better fit. Consider your daily habits and find moments where memory exercises can seamlessly integrate. Practice visualization techniques during a commute or use mnemonic devices while preparing meals. The key is to adapt exercises to become a natural part of your life rather than an added burden.

Tracking progress is an often overlooked yet vital part of memory improvement. Keeping a record of your achievements can boost motivation and provide tangible evidence of improvement. Simple tools like a journal or digital apps can help track your progress. Write down the exercises you complete, any challenges you face, and the successes you achieve. Regularly review these notes to identify trends and make informed adjustments to your routines. If a particular exercise isn't yielding results, don't hesitate to modify or replace it. Flexibility is essential, allowing you to adapt and optimize your strategies based on what works best for you.

The journey to improving memory is personal and ongoing. It's about building habits that support your goals and embracing a mindset open to change. By understanding your unique needs, setting realistic goals, and customizing exercises, you empower yourself to make meaningful progress. Regularly monitoring and adapting your approach ensures that your efforts remain practical and relevant. Remember that memory improvement is a gradual process, not a quick fix. It requires commitment and patience, but the rewards—a sharper mind, improved focus, and enhanced daily interactions—are worth the effort. Through these steps, you pave the way for a more vibrant and fulfilling cognitive experience.

CHAPTER TWO
LAYING THE FOUNDATION FOR COGNITIVE ENHANCEMENT

Imagine stepping into a room where everything you need is at your fingertips. The space is clear, organized, and inviting, with just enough light filtering through the windows. Now, think about how this environment might affect your ability to think, remember, and focus. Our surroundings profoundly impact our cognitive function, often in ways we don't immediately realize. This chapter delves into creating spaces that support memory and enhance your overall mental well-being. It's about turning your environment into an ally that encourages clarity and concentration.

A well-organized workspace is more than just aesthetically pleasing; it's a practical necessity for maintaining focus. Begin by decluttering your desk or office area. Remove unnecessary items that can distract you from the task at hand. Utilize storage solutions such as bins, trays, or shelves to keep essential items within reach but out of sight. A tidy space reduces cognitive load, allowing your mind to concentrate on what's important.

Additionally, consider using color and light to optimize your environment further. Soft, natural lighting can reduce eye strain and improve mood, while strategic pops of color can stimulate creativity and focus. Blues and greens, for instance, are known to have calming effects, which can enhance concentration and productivity.

Incorporating visual cues and reminders can significantly aid memory retention. Simple tools like sticky notes or index cards placed strategically around your workspace can serve as effective prompts for tasks or deadlines. Create a visual board where you can pin important dates, goals, or inspiring quotes. That keeps you organized and reinforces memory through repeated visual exposure. The more frequently you see these reminders, the more likely you are to remember them. This technique leverages the brain's natural inclination to notice and recall visual patterns, making it a powerful tool for memory enhancement.

Reducing cognitive load is crucial to maintaining focus throughout the day. Simplify your routines by establishing a consistent schedule that minimizes decision fatigue. Designate specific work, breaks, and leisure times to create a rhythm your mind can easily follow. Doing so frees up your mental resources for more critical thinking tasks. Decluttering your mental space is just as important as organizing your physical one. Consider using digital tools or apps to manage tasks and appointments, allowing you to offload information from your mind and reduce the mental clutter that can lead to fatigue.

LAYING THE FOUNDATION FOR COGNITIVE ENHANCEMENT 25

Interactive Element: Personalized Workspace Checklist

Take a moment to evaluate your current workspace. Use this checklist to identify areas for improvement:

- Are there unnecessary items on your desk that you can remove?
- Is the lighting comfortable for reading and working?
- Do you have visual reminders for essential tasks?
- Is there a designated place for frequently used items?

These prompts help you create a more conducive environment for memory and focus.

Creating a relaxing atmosphere is equally important in supporting memory and reducing stress. Integrate elements of nature into your space, such as plants or water features, which can promote a sense of calm and improve air quality. Studies have shown that even small interactions with nature can lower stress levels, enhancing cognitive performance. Aromatherapy is another effective method for creating a calming environment. Essential oils like lavender or rose have been found to reduce stress and anxiety, making them ideal for a workspace. According to a systematic review, over 70% of studies reported a positive effect on reducing stress and anxiety following aromatherapy interventions (SOURCE 1). Incorporating scents through diffusers or candles can create a soothing ambiance that supports better memory retention.

As you design your environment, remember that the goal is to create a space that works for you. It's about balancing order and inspiration, functionality and comfort. By optimizing your surroundings, you lay a strong foundation for cognitive enhancement, allowing you to focus more effectively, remember more clearly, and ultimately, live a more enriched life.

2.1 THE ROLE OF NUTRITION IN MEMORY IMPROVEMENT

What you eat plays a significant role in how well your brain functions. Essential nutrients fuel your cognitive engine, ensuring it runs smoothly and efficiently. Omega-3 fatty acids, found in foods like salmon, walnuts, and flaxseeds, are among these vital nutrients. They support brain health by improving cell membrane fluidity and enhancing neuron communication. This communication is integral for processes like memory and learning. Antioxidants, on the other hand, protect your brain from oxidative stress. Foods rich in antioxidants, such as berries, dark chocolate, and leafy greens, help neutralize free radicals, thus preserving your cognitive functions.

Dietary patterns also influence your mental acuity. The Mediterranean diet, known for its emphasis on fruits, vegetables, whole grains, and healthy fats, is particularly beneficial. Research indicates that this diet is associated with a lower risk of cognitive decline and improved memory performance. The diet's richness in omega-3s, antioxidants, and anti-inflammatory properties creates an environment that supports brain health. Adopting such a dietary pattern gives your brain a balanced mix of nutrients that bolsters cognitive resilience and longevity.

Hydration is another crucial component of cognitive performance. The brain comprises nearly 75% water, so that slight dehydration can impair its functions. Symptoms of dehydration include headaches, fatigue, and, notably, memory lapses. To maintain mental clarity, aim to drink enough water throughout the day. Water intake needs can vary, but a general guideline is to consume around eight glasses daily. Remember, thirst is a late indicator of dehydration, so it's wise to drink regularly, even if you don't feel thirsty.

While focusing on what to consume for optimal brain health, it's equally important to recognize and avoid dietary pitfalls. High sugar intake can negatively affect brain functions by disrupting insulin regulation and increasing inflammation. This impact can lead to memory problems and slower cognitive processing. Limiting sugary snacks and beverages can help maintain stable blood sugar levels, which improves brain health. Processed foods laden with unhealthy fats and additives also risk cognitive function. Regular consumption can lead to inflammation and oxidative stress, both detrimental to memory. Opting for whole, unprocessed foods over convenience meals can make a significant difference in maintaining a sharp mind.

Visual Element: Brain-Boosting Foods Infographic

Create an infographic highlighting the top brain-boosting foods, such as salmon, berries, and nuts. Include their key benefits and how they support memory and cognition. This visual guide can serve as a quick reference for planning brain-healthy meals.

Understanding the role of nutrition in memory improvement empowers you to make informed choices about your diet. You can enhance your cognitive function and preserve your memory by incorporating brain-boosting nutrients, following beneficial dietary patterns, staying hydrated, and avoiding harmful foods.

2.2 MINDFULNESS AS A TOOL FOR BETTER FOCUS

In a world buzzing with constant activity, mindfulness offers a refuge of calm and clarity. At its core, mindfulness is about embracing the present moment with full awareness and without judgment. It's a practice that encourages you to pay attention to what's happening right now rather than getting lost in thoughts of the past or future. This focus on the present can significantly enhance cognitive function by reducing mental clutter and improving concentration. When you are mindful, you create a mental space to process information more clearly and effectively, which is particularly beneficial for those seeking to improve memory.

You can practice mindfulness through various exercises that directly bolster memory and concentration. One effective technique is mindful breathing, where you focus solely on the rhythm of your breath. As you inhale and exhale, allow each breath to anchor you in the moment, clearing your mind of distractions. This simple act can enhance mental clarity, making absorbing and recalling information easier. Another valuable exercise is the body scan meditation. It involves mentally scanning each part of your body, from head to toe, and tuning into the sensations you feel. This practice heightens awareness and helps you connect more deeply with your physical presence, fostering a stronger mind-body connection that aids memory retention.

Incorporating mindfulness into your daily life doesn't require significant changes to your routine. It can be as simple as practicing mindful eating, where you focus all your senses on the experience of eating. Pay attention to your food's texture, flavor, and aroma, and notice how these details enhance your sensory memory. Walking meditation offers another opportunity to integrate mindfulness into everyday activities. As you walk, bring awareness to each step, the sensation of your feet touching the ground, and the rhythm of your movement. This practice improves concentration and transforms routine walks into opportunities for mental refreshment.

Regular mindfulness practice brings many cognitive benefits that extend beyond improved memory. One of the most significant advantages is stress reduction. By fostering a sense of calm and presence, mindfulness helps lower stress levels, which can otherwise impair memory and cognitive function. Over time, sustained mindfulness practice can lead to enhanced emotional regulation, allowing you to respond to life's challenges with more remarkable composure and clarity. This emotional balance contributes to better focus and decision-making, as you're less likely to be overwhelmed by stress or distracted by negative emotions.

Interactive Element: Mindfulness Practice Tracker

Consider using a simple tracker to monitor your mindfulness practice. Note the exercises you practice daily, their duration, and any observations or feelings. Over time, this tracker can help you identify patterns and see progress in your mindfulness and cognitive improvements.

Mindfulness is a powerful tool for cognitive enhancement, offering a pathway to sharpen focus and improve memory. By integrating mindfulness into your daily routine, you cultivate an environment of mental clarity and reduced stress. These practices support better cognitive function and enhance your overall quality of life. As you explore mindfulness, remember that consistency is critical. The benefits grow with regular practice, leading to a more focused, resilient mind.

Life is an ever-changing journey that we constantly try to keep up. Our bodies change, our minds change, and our routines change. So how do we keep up? It's true that when we're young, we may be able to keep up with the pace of life, but as we age, we can't quite keep up anymore. Our bodies become sore, and our memories fade. But we can keep our memories if we work hard enough.

In the world of memory, you'll find that everything is connected. We often forget this, but it's an important thing we need to keep in mind. That is why staying mentally sharp is so important. We need to keep sharp to remember the things we love, the things we've lost, and the things we've learned. But how do we stay sharp? We must take care of our minds as we do our bodies. We cannot let them become weak, or they'll fade away.

Our brains comprise neurons that work together to help us learn and remember information. The neurons in our brains communicate and are connected through these networks, which work together to help us learn and remember information. When working to learn something new, it's important to remember that the best way to do so is through practice because we are creatures of habit.

The phrase "practice makes perfect" is not new, yet it still holds. While it may be difficult to see how different habits can impact our lives, it is essential to understand that they do. Remembering that we create a new memory every time we perform a task is good. This memory creates a pattern in our brain, which allows us to remember things and how to do them. The more we do this, the better we become at it, which is why it is so important to practice.

Many have heard the phrase "use it or lose it." That is a term often used about the brain. As we age, our brains become less efficient, and we lose our ability to do certain things. That is because we are not using our brains, and they are not getting the necessary exercise. One of the main reasons why it is so important to exercise our minds is that they are the most valuable things we have.

One of the best ways to keep our minds sharp is to keep learning. We must continue learning, even if we're not in school. We should keep our minds active by learning new things and challenging ourselves. The more we know, the more we will be able to do and the more we will be able to remember.

Another way to keep our minds sharp is to practice meditation. It is one of the most effective ways, as it allows us to focus and relax. Meditation is a great way to relieve stress and help us focus on the things that matter most.

It is important to remember that we are not alone. Many people are going through the same things as us, and they are going through it, too. We are not alone, and we will get through this together. We must remember that we are not alone and are not the only ones going through this.

Ultimately, it is essential to remember that we are not alone. We are on this journey together and will get through it together. We must remember that we are not alone and are not the only ones going through this. We are all in this together and will get through it together.

2.3 SETTING ACHIEVABLE MEMORY IMPROVEMENT GOALS

Picture this: you're at the starting line of a race, but instead of a clear path, you have a maze of possibilities, each more overwhelming than the last. That is often how memory improvement can feel without a clear set of goals. Setting specific, achievable goals is crucial because it transforms this overwhelming maze into a guided path. It acts as a motivational tool, offering a sense of direction and purpose. When you set a goal, you give yourself a target, something tangible to aim for. This focus helps maintain motivation, especially when progress seems slow or challenging.

Enter the concept of SMART goals, a framework designed to create clear and attainable objectives. SMART stands for Specific, Measurable, Achievable, Relevant, and Time-bound. Applying this to memory exercises means setting clearly defined and trackable goals. For instance, instead of saying, "I want to remember more," a SMART goal would be, "I will memorize the names of three new people each week for the next month." This specific target clarifies what you're aiming for and provides a way to measure success. By ensuring that your goals are achievable and relevant, you set yourself up for victory. Time-bound goals add an element of urgency, encouraging consistent effort and focus.

Monitoring your progress is as important as setting the goals themselves. Tracking allows you to see how far you've come and where you might need to adjust your approach. Several tools can aid this process, from simple journals to digital apps designed for cognitive improvement. These tools can help you log daily activities, note challenges, and celebrate victories. Flexibility is vital; be prepared to adjust your goals as you progress. If you find a particular exercise isn't working as well as expected, tweak your approach or set a new target. This adaptability aligns your efforts with your current abilities and needs, ensuring continuous progress.

Celebrating milestones is a vital part of maintaining motivation and engagement. Each small achievement is a step forward, a testament to your hard work and dedication. Acknowledging these moments in a personal journal can provide a record of your journey, offering encouragement on more challenging days. Consider implementing a reward system for meeting specific cognitive milestones. Rewards don't have to be extravagant; they can be simple treats or activities you enjoy. This positive reinforcement boosts morale and reinforces the behavior, making it more likely you'll continue striving toward your goals.

As you set out on this path of memory improvement, remember that goals are your guideposts. They provide clarity and direction, helping you navigate the complexities of cognitive enhancement. By setting SMART goals, tracking your progress, and celebrating achievements, you lay a strong foundation for sustained improvement. This chapter has laid the groundwork for building an effective memory improvement strategy. Next, we'll explore the practical exercises that will bring these goals to life, offering actionable steps to enhance memory and cognitive function.

CHAPTER THREE
PROVEN MEMORY ENHANCEMENT TECHNIQUES

Imagine walking through your childhood home. Each room holds vivid memories, from joyous moments to everyday routines. You can see the worn-out carpet, feel the coolness of the kitchen tiles, and even smell the faint aroma of your favorite meal cooking. This ability to recall details by mentally navigating familiar spaces is the essence of the Memory Palace technique, a powerful tool for enhancing memory. The Memory Palace, or method of loci, has long been employed by memory champions to recall vast amounts of information, leveraging the strength of our spatial memory. This method taps into our natural ability to remember locations and uses it to associate those spaces with information we wish to recall. It transforms abstract data into concrete images placed within a familiar spatial context, making retrieval more intuitive.

The Memory Palace technique dates back to ancient Greece and Rome, where orators like Cicero used it to deliver long speeches without notes. They would visualize a familiar building, assigning each speech point to specific locations. They could easily recall each discourse segment by mentally walking through the building. This technique relies on the brain's robust spatial memory, which is less prone to interference than other types of memory. The process involves memorizing a layout, such as your home, and associating each item to remember with a specific locus within that layout. For example, you might place the first item in the living room and the next in the kitchen. Later, retrieval is achieved by mentally walking through these loci, allowing each location to cue the desired memories (SOURCE 1).

Creating your own Memory Palace begins with selecting a space you know well. Your home is ideal, as its layout is already etched into your memory. Alternatively, consider using your workplace or another location you frequently visit. The key is to choose a space you can visualize in detail, as these details will serve as anchors for the information you wish to remember. Once you've selected your space, mentally divide it into distinct loci or points of interest. These could be rooms, specific pieces of furniture, or noteworthy landmarks within the space. At each locus, place a piece of information you want to recall. For instance, assign each key point to a different room if you're memorizing a speech. Visualize the point interacting with the features of that room, creating a vivid mental image that links the information to the location.

The effectiveness of the Memory Palace hinges on your ability to visualize clearly, so cultivating visualization skills is essential. Begin with daily mental walk-throughs of your chosen space. As you move from room to room, practice recalling the information associated with each locus. Visualization drills, like focusing on the minor details of a familiar object or scene, can enhance your ability to retain intricate images. These exercises train your brain to notice and remember delicate information, improving the vividness of your mental pictures. Over time, these practices will strengthen the neural pathways involved in visualization, making recalling information stored within your Memory Palace more accessible.

The applications of the Memory Palace are vast and varied. Whether trying to remember a grocery list or preparing for an exam, this technique can be a game-changer. For lists, assign each item to a different locus, visualizing an exaggerated interaction between the item and the location. To prepare for a presentation, break your content into crucial points and assign each end to a locus. Each location will trigger the associated information as you walk through your Memory Palace. The technique is instrumental when dealing with complex or voluminous data, as it efficiently organizes and retrieves information.

Interactive Element: Building Your Memory Palace

Create a map of your chosen Memory Palace. Mark each locus with what you want to remember. As you practice, update the map with new loci and information. This visual aid will reinforce your mental images and support your memory exercise.

Integrating the Memory Palace technique into your routine can unlock new potential in your memory abilities. This method enhances recall and offers a structured way to manage and retrieve information, helping you navigate the complexities of daily life with greater ease and confidence.

3.1 MNEMONICS: CRAFTING EFFECTIVE MEMORY AIDS

When you think of mnemonics, imagine them as mental shortcuts designed to make remembering easier. They are clever tools that help bridge the gap between forgetfulness and recall, acting like a string tied around your finger to remind you of something important. These cognitive shortcuts transform complex information into simple cues, making it easier to retrieve from memory. Whether it's remembering a grocery list, a set of numbers, or historical dates, mnemonics provide a structured approach to recall by leveraging patterns and associations your brain naturally understands.

There are various types of mnemonics, each suited to different kinds of information. Acronyms, for instance, turn multiple words into a single memorable word. Take ROYGBIV, which stands for the colors of the rainbow—red, orange, yellow, green, blue, indigo, violet. Rhymes are another mnemonic device, ideal for remembering facts or dates. For example, the rhyme "In fourteen hundred ninety-two, Columbus sailed the ocean blue" helps us recall the year of Columbus's voyage. Visual imagery associations take things further by linking complex concepts with vivid images. Imagine trying to remember a complex biological process by picturing it as a lively cartoon scene, where each character represents a step in the process. These images stick because the brain loves stories and pictures.

Creating personalized mnemonics tailors these tools to fit your unique memory style. Start by connecting new information to your interests or experiences. For example, if you're passionate about music, use song lyrics to encode a list of tasks. Incorporating humor or vivid imagery can also make mnemonics more effective. If you're trying to memorize a list of ingredients, imagine them in a silly scenario—like a tomato juggling onions while wearing a cheese hat. The more absurd, the better, as these exaggerated images are less likely to blend into the mundane and more likely to be remembered.

Integrating mnemonics into your learning routine can transform how you retain information. In language learning, mnemonics can help memorize vocabulary by associating foreign words with similar-sounding words in your native language. For historical data or scientific terms, crafting a narrative or visual story around the information can make it more engaging and memorable. For instance, if you're learning about the elements of the periodic table, visualize a comic strip where each element is a superhero with distinct powers. These narratives make learning more enjoyable and enhance retention by embedding information into a structured storyline.

Interactive Element: Mnemonic Creation Exercise

Take a list of five items you need to memorize. Create a personalized mnemonic for each item using acronyms, rhymes, or visual imagery. Reflect on which mnemonic type feels most natural and effective for you, noting your preferences in a journal for future reference.

Using mnemonics involves tapping into the brain's love for patterns and associations. These tools simplify recall, making abstract information tangible and easy to grasp. As you incorporate them into your study routine, you likely find that recalling details becomes smoother and more intuitive, freeing up mental space for new learning.

3.2 CHUNKING INFORMATION FOR EASIER RECALL

Have you ever noticed how easy it is to remember your phone number when broken into chunks? This technique, chunking, is a powerful tool for enhancing memory retention by simplifying complex information. Chunking involves grouping related information into manageable units, making it easier for your brain to process and recall. Organizing data into smaller, meaningful segments reduces cognitive load, allowing your mind to store and retrieve information more efficiently. Chunking capitalizes on our brain's natural tendency to seek patterns and associations, turning an overwhelming amount of information into something digestible. This cognitive strategy can transform how you approach learning and memory tasks, providing a structured way to handle information overload.

In practical terms, chunking can aid memory across various context memory. Consider how you break down a long phone number or ID code. Instead of trying to remember a string of ten digits, you divide it into smaller groups, like 123-456-7890. That simplifies the task and aligns with how our memory systems naturally function. Similarly, when studying, organizing material into thematic sections can vastly improve comprehension and recall. For instance, if you're learning about world history, you might chunk information by periods or geographical regions. This method allows you to focus on one section at a time, reinforcing connections between related concepts and facilitating a deeper understanding of the material. By framing information to mirror the brain's natural processing, chunking helps embed it more firmly into long-term memory.

In everyday life, chunking proves invaluable for managing tasks and processing information. When planning your daily schedule, try grouping similar activities. You could dedicate time to all your work-related tasks, followed by a chunk for personal errands. Organizing your day into chunks minimizes the mental effort required to switch between tasks, enhancing productivity and focus. Shopping lists provide another opportunity to apply chunking. Instead of haphazardly jotting down items, categorize them by store section—produce, dairy, pantry items. This approach speeds up your shopping trip and makes it easier to remember everything you need. Chunking simplifies complex tasks, allowing you to approach them clearly and efficiently.

To enhance your chunking skills, start with exercises that challenge your short-term memory. Engage in games that require you to recall sequences or patterns, such as memory card games or number puzzles. These activities train your brain to recognize and organize information quickly, honing your ability to create meaningful chunks. Pattern recognition exercises, like sorting objects based on shared characteristics, further develop your chunking prowess. Practicing these skills regularly strengthens your cognitive efficiency, making it second nature to group and recall information in your daily life. With time and dedication, chunking becomes a seamless part of your memory strategy, empowering you to tackle information with confidence and ease.

3.3 THE POWER OF REPETITION AND SPACING EFFECT

Memory thrives on repetition, a fundamental principle that reinforces what we learn. Think about how children learn the alphabet through repeated exposure: sing the song enough times, and it sticks. This concept isn't limited to childhood learning; it spans our lives. Repetition solidifies our connection to the material, embedding it deeply into our memory. But repetition alone isn't the whole story. The spacing effect, a robust phenomenon, reveals that spreading learning sessions over time enhances retention far more than cramming information in one go. Hermann Ebbinghaus, a pioneering figure in memory research, discovered that memory significantly improves when learning occurs at spaced intervals. This approach, known as spaced repetition, optimizes long-term retention by allowing time for the brain to consolidate information between sessions.

Designing an effective repetition schedule requires thoughtful planning, considering both the nature of the material and your personal goals. For language learning, daily review sessions can be particularly beneficial. By revisiting vocabulary daily, you maintain a steady rhythm that reinforces your grasp of new words. Similarly, for professional skills, incorporating weekly refreshers can help keep knowledge sharp and relevant. That could involve weekly time to revisit critical concepts or practice specific skills. The key is consistency. Establishing a routine that integrates regular review into your schedule creates a sustainable framework for reinforcing memory. This structured approach minimizes the likelihood of forgetting, transforming learning into a more manageable and rewarding process.

Fortunately, technology offers numerous tools to facilitate spaced repetition, making integrating this technique into your daily life easier. Apps like Anki and Quizlet are explicitly designed for this purpose, allowing you to create digital flashcards that prompt you to review material optimally. These apps take the guesswork out of scheduling, using algorithms to determine when to revisit each card based on your performance. Manual-spaced repetition planning can also be effective for those who prefer a more hands-on approach. That could involve using a calendar to track review sessions or creating a physical system of flashcards organized by review frequency. Whether digital or manual, the goal is to establish a consistent pattern of review that aligns with your learning objectives.

Balancing repetition with rest is crucial to avoid cognitive overload and ensure effective memory consolidation. Sleep, often underestimated, plays a significant role in this process. During sleep, the brain processes and organizes information from the day, strengthening neural connections that underpin memory. Ensuring you get enough rest is vital for maximizing the benefits of repetition. Structured breaks, too, are essential. They allow your mind to rejuvenate, preventing burnout and keeping you fresh for future learning sessions. By alternating periods of focused review with rest intervals, you create an environment that supports cognitive health and memory enhancement. This balance allows you to maintain momentum without succumbing to the fatigue that can accompany intensive study, ensuring that your efforts in repetition translate into meaningful and lasting improvements in memory.

3.4 LEVERAGING STORYTELLING TO ENHANCE MEMORY

Storytelling is an ancient art deeply rooted in human culture and used to pass down knowledge and experiences. This method engages multiple cognitive processes, making it a powerful tool for memory enhancement. When you hear a story, your brain doesn't just listen; it visualizes, empathizes, and predicts, activating areas related to language, sensory perception, and emotion. This multisensory engagement is why stories stick with us longer than dry facts. They create a rich tapestry where information is woven into a narrative, making it easier for the brain to recall. Stories transform abstract data into something tangible and relatable by appealing to emotions and creating vivid mental images. This transformation not only aids recall but also enhances understanding as you process information in a way that resonates on a personal level.

Crafting memorable stories around the information you wish to remember can be incredibly effective. Start by incorporating characters and plots into your learning material. Imagine trying to memorize historical events by turning them into a story with protagonists, conflicts, and resolutions. This strategy allows you to engage with the material more deeply and remember details more easily. Using metaphors and analogies can simplify abstract concepts, making them more accessible. For instance, you might compare complex scientific processes to a familiar scenario, like a day at the beach, where each process element corresponds to a part of the experience. This comparison helps anchor new information to existing knowledge, facilitating easier recall.

In educational and professional settings, storytelling proves invaluable. Case studies serve as practical examples, illustrating theoretical concepts in a real-world context. When studying a case, you follow a narrative demonstrating how certain principles apply, making learning more dynamic and memorable. Similarly, narrative techniques can convey organizational values or strategies through compelling stories during corporate training. You ensure the information is retained and internalized by embedding lessons in narratives. This internalization is crucial for applying knowledge effectively, as it fosters a deeper connection to the material, inspiring more intuitive and informed decision-making.

Personalizing stories is a crucial aspect of maximizing their mnemonic potential. Personal anecdotes around historical events or technical subjects make the content more relevant and engaging. Think of a time you learned best through an individual experience. Visualizing historical events as if you were part of them or imagining technical subjects within a familiar context creates a personalized framework that enhances recall. This approach allows you to use your unique perspective and experiences to enrich the learning process, making it more enjoyable and effective.

Improving your storytelling skills can further bolster your memory outcomes. Practice creative writing exercises to hone your ability to construct engaging narratives. These exercises encourage you to think critically about structure, pacing, and detail, all contributing to more compelling stories. Consider joining storytelling workshops or clubs where you can learn from others and refine your craft. Engaging with a community of storytellers provides feedback and inspiration, helping you develop your skills in a supportive environment. This development not only aids in memory enhancement but also enriches your communication abilities, enabling you to convey ideas more clearly and persuasively.

As we draw this chapter to a close, remember that the techniques discussed—whether visualizing with the Memory Palace, using mnemonics, chunking, repetition, or storytelling—are tools to empower your memory. These methods aren't just about remembering facts but transforming how you interact with information. They offer pathways to deeper understanding and better retention. In the next chapter, we'll explore practical exercises to integrate these techniques into daily life, building a robust foundation for cognitive enhancement.

CHAPTER FOUR
PRACTICAL DAILY EXERCISES FOR MEMORY BOOST

Imagine waking up each morning with clarity and readiness, your mind sharp and eager to tackle the day ahead. You can improve the state of cognitive alertness through a thoughtfully designed morning routine that prioritizes activities to enhance your memory. The morning hours offer a unique opportunity to set the tone for the entire day. As the world begins to stir, your brain is particularly receptive to exercises that stimulate mental agility and reinforce memory retention. By engaging in routine morning practices, you can create a foundation of mental resilience that carries through the day's challenges.

Starting your day with cognitive exercises can significantly enhance your alertness and memory. The rhythm of morning routines profoundly impacts cognitive readiness, priming your mind for the tasks ahead. Just as athletes warm up before a race, your brain benefits from a routine that boosts cognitive functions. Incorporating simple exercises into your morning can sharpen your focus and boost your memory. Activities like crossword puzzles or Sudoku are excellent for mental agility. These puzzles challenge your brain, encouraging it to think critically and solve problems, which can improve overall cognitive function. Similarly, memory recall games, such as listing items or tasks from memory, strengthen your ability to retrieve information, a skill that becomes increasingly important as the day progresses.

Visualization techniques provide another layer of cognitive preparation, allowing you to mentally organize and anticipate the day's activities. Spend a few moments visualizing your schedule or goals for the day. Picture each task in detail, imagining the steps needed to accomplish it. This mental rehearsal prepares you for the day and strengthens neural pathways associated with planning and execution. Visualization can transform abstract tasks into concrete actions, making it easier to approach the day with confidence and clarity.

Pairing cognitive exercises with physical activity creates a holistic approach to morning routines. Physical activity boosts brain power by increasing blood flow and promoting neuroplasticity, the brain's ability to adapt and grow. Consider incorporating a morning walk with mindful reflection. As you walk, focus on the sensations around you— the sound of birds, the feel of the breeze, the rhythm of your steps. This practice invigorates your body and centers your mind, preparing you to face the day with renewed focus. Stretching routines paired with mental affirmations can also be effective. As you stretch, repeat affirmations that reinforce your goals and aspirations. This combination of physical and psychological engagement sets a positive tone, enhancing your mood and cognitive readiness.

Interactive Element: Morning Routine Checklist

Create a checklist of morning activities that enhance cognitive function. Include puzzles or games, visualization exercises, and physical activities. Use this checklist to track your weekly routine, noting how these practices influence your memory and alertness.

By embracing a morning routine rich with cognitive exercises, you lay the groundwork for a day of heightened focus and improved memory. These practices boost your mental agility and cultivate a sense of preparedness and resilience. As you integrate these exercises into your routine, you'll likely find that your days begin with greater clarity and purpose, empowering you to navigate challenges confidently and quickly.

4.1 LUNCHTIME NEUROBICS: BREAK ROUTINE WITH COGNITIVE WORKOUTS

Imagine pausing in the middle of a hectic day, taking a moment to refresh your mind and recharge your energy. This power of a midday break is often underestimated. When you break away from routine, especially with activities designed to stimulate your brain, you prevent cognitive fatigue and enhance productivity for the rest of the day. Neurobic exercises—simple yet effective—are perfect for such breaks. They target different areas of your brain, keeping it agile and alert. These exercises create a mental oasis that rejuvenates and prepares you for the afternoon's challenges. This strategic pause is not just a break; it boosts your cognitive capabilities, ensuring your mind remains sharp and focused.

Even a brief foray into neurobic exercises can work wonders for your cognitive state during lunch. Start with using your non-dominant hand for routine tasks like writing or eating. This simple switch challenges your brain, activating pathways that aren't typically engaged and promoting greater flexibility in thinking. Solving brain teasers or logic puzzles is another excellent option. These puzzles stimulate your problem-solving abilities and require you to think critically, which enhances overall cognitive function. Consider introducing variety to maintain interest—one day, tackle a crossword, and the next, try a Sudoku puzzle. This diversity keeps your brain guessing and growing, preventing monotony and ensuring continuous engagement.

Incorporating sensory activities into your lunchtime routine can further enhance brain activity. Our senses are powerful tools for memory and cognition. Engage them by exploring new flavors or spices during your meal. This act makes eating more enjoyable and stimulates your taste and smell senses, closely linked to memory. Try a new fruit or spice, and focus on the experience—the aroma, taste, and texture. This sensory engagement can create vivid memories, enriching your cognitive landscape. It's a delightful way to turn an everyday activity into a meaningful cognitive exercise, with the benefit of expanding your culinary horizons.

Engaging with colleagues in collaborative cognitive activities can transform the workplace into a supportive environment for mental growth. Group memory games or trivia challenges are perfect for lunch breaks. These activities foster camaraderie and provide a fun, competitive edge that encourages everyone to participate. They also tap into social dynamics, which are essential for cognitive health. Working together on problem-solving exercises can enhance creativity and build team spirit. When you solve problems as a team, you benefit from diverse perspectives, which can lead to innovative solutions. This collaborative approach strengthens individual cognition and enhances collective problem-solving skills.

Interactive Element: Lunchtime Neurobics Challenge

Create a weekly challenge with colleagues to try different neurobic exercises during lunch breaks. Rotate responsibilities for selecting activities and keeping the experience fresh and engaging. Document your experiences and reflections in a shared journal, noting any improvements in focus or creativity throughout the week.

Incorporating these activities into your lunch break transforms a simple pause into an opportunity for cognitive enhancement. As you explore different exercises, you'll likely discover which resonates most with you and bring the most significant benefit. This approach ensures that your midday break is a time for rest and a chance to rejuvenate your mind, preparing you for whatever the afternoon may bring.

4.2 EVENING REFLECTION: CONSOLIDATING DAILY LEARNING

As the day winds down, there's a unique opportunity to engage in evening reflection. That is not just a moment to unwind but a crucial practice for consolidating the day's experiences and learnings. Reflection acts as a bridge between short-term experiences and long-term memory. By taking time to think about the events of your day, you reinforce neural pathways, making it easier to retain information. This process can transform fleeting moments into lasting memories, providing a rich tapestry of experiences to draw from. Evening reflection creates a space for mindfulness, where you can assess what you've learned, identify areas for improvement, and appreciate the day's achievements. In this quiet time, your mind can process the day's events, turning over new ideas and solidifying them in your memory.

One powerful tool for evening reflection is journaling. This practice encourages you to articulate your thoughts and experiences, providing a tangible record of your day. Writing about critical events or learnings serves as a powerful reinforcement for memory. It helps organize your thoughts, clarifying what you've experienced and learned. This clarity contributes to a deeper understanding and better recall. Gratitude journaling can add a positive dimension to this reflection. By noting things you're grateful for, you shift your focus to positive experiences, which can improve mood and mental well-being. This practice encourages a more optimistic outlook, reinforcing positive memories while reducing stress and anxiety. Keeping a journal becomes a record of your days and a tool for personal growth and cognitive enhancement.

Meditation and relaxation techniques are invaluable in winding down at the end of the day. They create a peaceful transition from the busyness of daily life to rest and recovery. Guided meditation sessions focusing on the day's highlights can help you relax and reflect. As you meditate, allow your mind to revisit significant moments, acknowledging their impact and letting go of any associated stress. This practice not only supports mental calmness but also enhances memory consolidation. The relaxed state achieved through meditation encourages deeper processing of information, improving retention and recall. Relaxation techniques, such as deep breathing or progressive muscle relaxation, further support this process by creating a tranquil environment where the mind can unwind and recharge.

Reviewing and rehearsing information learned during the day is another effective method for strengthening memory retention. That can involve reviewing notes or lessons from your daily activities, reinforcing what you've learned. By revisiting information, you help solidify it in your mind, making it easier to recall in the future. This practice benefits students or professionals who need to retain large amounts of information. It transforms learning from passive to active, where you engage with the material repeatedly, deepening your understanding. Whether reviewing academic material, work-related tasks, or personal insights, this end-of-day review ensures that your learning is accessible and usable.

Visual Element: Reflection and Rehearsal Guide

Create a simple guide outlining steps for evening reflection and rehearsal. Include sections for journaling prompts, meditation techniques, and review strategies. Use this guide to structure your evening routine, ensuring a comprehensive approach to memory consolidation.

4.3 WEEKEND MEMORY CHALLENGES: FUN EXERCISES FOR FAMILIES

Involving family members in memory improvement activities transforms the process into a shared experience, fostering deeper connections and creating lasting memories. Engaging in such activities as a family strengthens cognitive abilities and enhances emotional bonds. Shared challenges and successes create a supportive environment where everyone feels valued and encouraged. Families work together toward a common goal, such as improving memory and developing a sense of unity and teamwork. These activities offer a unique opportunity for cognitive bonding, where members contribute their strengths and learn from one another. This collaborative approach makes memory exercises enjoyable and meaningful, turning them into cherished family traditions.

Interactive memory games are a fantastic way for families to spend time together while enhancing their cognitive skills. Imagine gathering around the living room table for a spirited game of Concentration. As each card is flipped, laughter and excitement fill the air. This classic game challenges players to recall matching pairs' positions, exercising short-term and working memory. By playing regularly, families can see improvements in attention and recall, all while having fun. Another engaging option is storytelling games, where each person adds a sentence to a developing plot. This activity stretches the imagination and requires players to remember previous contributions, building a coherent and entertaining narrative. These games encourage creativity, improve language skills, and strengthen memory, making them a perfect activity for family weekends.

Outdoor activities offer a refreshing change of pace, combining physical exercise with memory challenges. Consider organizing a scavenger hunt with memory clues. As family members dash around the yard or park, they search for hidden items based on riddles or hints. This activity promotes problem-solving, critical thinking, and teamwork while providing a healthy dose of physical activity. Participants must remember clues and locations, engaging both their minds and bodies. Nature walks present another excellent opportunity for outdoor memory exercises. As you stroll through a nearby park or nature reserve, challenge family members to identify plants, animals, or landmarks. This activity encourages observation and recall, enhancing memory through interaction with the natural world.

Creative projects offer yet another avenue for cognitive engagement and memory enhancement. Consider setting aside a weekend afternoon for a family photo collage project. Gather photos from family events, vacations, and everyday moments, and work together to arrange them into a collage. As you create the collage, discuss the stories behind each photo, adding captions or anecdotes. This exercise stimulates creativity and reinforces memories through storytelling and reflection. Building a scrapbook is a similar project you can do over several weekends. Encourage each family member to contribute entries, recounting personal experiences or highlighting special occasions. As the scrapbook grows, it becomes a tangible record of shared memories, reinforcing the connections between family members and the events that shaped their lives.

4.4 TRACKING PROGRESS: HOW TO MEASURE YOUR MEMORY IMPROVEMENT

Progress tracking is a powerful motivator. Seeing tangible improvements can fuel your commitment and drive as you enhance your memory. When you track your progress, you record your journey—each small victory, each hurdle overcome. This record not only provides proof of your efforts but also acts as a reminder of your capabilities and potential. Knowing where you began and how far you've come can be incredibly encouraging, especially on days when motivation wanes. By regularly monitoring your progress, you will focus on the goals and thus ensure that your efforts remain aligned with the desired outcomes.

Various methods exist to track cognitive improvement, offering unique insights into your progress. A memory improvement journal is one such tool. This journal serves as a personal log where you can record daily activities, exercises, and reflections. By jotting down your experiences, you create a comprehensive overview of your memory practices and their effects. This record lets you identify patterns and trends, highlighting the most effective exercises.

Additionally, digital apps designed for cognitive tracking can complement your journal. These apps offer features like reminders, progress charts, and performance assessments, providing a structured way to monitor your improvement. Combining these methods gives you a holistic view of your memory journey, empowering you to make informed decisions about your practices.

Setting benchmarks and milestones is another crucial aspect of progress tracking. These markers provide specific targets to aim for, giving your efforts direction and purpose. Start by establishing clear milestones for your memory exercises. These could be as simple as memorizing a new list of words each week or improving your recall speed for specific tasks. By breaking your larger goals into smaller, achievable milestones, you create a roadmap for success. Each milestone reached offers a sense of accomplishment, reinforcing your commitment to your goals. Tracking these milestones boosts your confidence and provides a tangible measure of your progress, keeping you motivated and engaged.

Evaluating the effectiveness of your exercises is essential to optimize your memory gains. Regular reflection on your practices allows you to assess which techniques yield the best results. Take time to consider how different exercises impact your memory. Are there specific activities that consistently lead to noticeable improvements? Conversely, are there exercises that seem less effective? By evaluating these factors, you can adapt your routines to better suit your needs. This flexibility ensures that your efforts remain productive, preventing stagnation and maximizing cognitive enhancement. Adjusting your strategies based on these reflections enhances your ability to achieve your memory goals.

As you track your progress, remember that the path to memory improvement is sometimes linear. There may be fluctuations in your performance, and that's okay. The key is to remain consistent and adaptable, using progress tracking to guide your efforts. You create a dynamic and responsive memory improvement plan by staying committed to your goals and regularly evaluating your practices. This approach fosters continuous growth, allowing you to build a stronger, more resilient memory.

When you track your progress, you create a narrative of your cognitive growth that celebrates milestones and adapts to challenges. Progress tracking keeps you focused and motivated, providing the insight to optimize your memory practices. As you integrate these tracking methods into your routine, you lay the foundation for sustained cognitive enhancement. With each step forward, you move closer to unlocking your full memory potential.

CHAPTER FIVE
ADAPTING EXERCISES TO YOUR COGNITIVE LEVEL

Imagine standing at the base of a mountain, looking up at the summit. The climb seems daunting, but you know the view from the top will be worth it. Memory improvement is much like this climb. It starts with small, simple steps that gradually build your confidence and ability. Just as a climber begins by tackling easy trails, you can embark on your memory enhancement journey with beginner exercises that seamlessly integrate into your daily life. These foundational exercises are designed to be approachable and practical, setting the stage for more advanced techniques as you progress.

One of the most straightforward ways to enhance your memory is through basic recall activities using everyday objects. Consider the items you interact with daily—keys, a wallet, or even a coffee mug. Try placing these objects in new locations daily, and then challenge yourself to remember where you put them. This simple exercise engages your brain in encoding and retrieval, reinforcing your ability to recall information. Similarly, word association games with everyday items can be fun and beneficial. Take a book, for instance, and think of a word that starts with each letter of its title. This activity sparks creativity and strengthens neural connections by encouraging your brain to explore new associations.

Building confidence in your memory capabilities can be both rewarding and enjoyable. Memory games provide a playful yet effective means of boosting your cognitive skills. Match-the-pair card games, for example, require you to remember the location of matching cards, honing your attention and recall. As you flip each card, your brain works to retain the images and their positions, enhancing your short-term memory. Alphabet memory challenges offer another engaging option. Try recalling words that start with each letter of the alphabet, or create a story using sequential letters. These exercises stimulate mental agility and expand your vocabulary, providing a solid foundation for more complex memory tasks.

Incorporating accessible practices into your daily routine can further enhance your memory. One such practice is daily journaling of crucial events. At the end of each day, take a few minutes to jot down memorable moments or new information you encountered. This habit not only reinforces memory retention but also promotes reflection and mindfulness. Another effective technique is using mnemonic rhymes for shared lists. Creating a catchy rhyme can make it easier to remember, whether a shopping list or a set of errands. These rhymes act as mental hooks, providing a structured way to retain information with minimal effort.

Evaluating your progress as a beginner is crucial to maintaining motivation without feeling overwhelmed. Start by tracking small achievements in a memory journal. Record the exercises you complete, noting any improvements or challenges. This practice allows you to see tangible evidence of your growth, reinforcing your commitment to memory enhancement. Celebrating consistency in training is equally important. Acknowledge your dedication by maintaining a routine, and reward yourself for reaching milestones, no matter how small. This positive reinforcement encourages continued effort, fostering a sense of accomplishment and motivation.

Interactive Element: Memory Progress Tracker

Create a simple progress tracker to monitor your memory exercises. Include columns for the date, exercise type, duration, and observations or reflections. This tracker can visually represent your journey, highlighting your achievements and guiding future practice.

By embracing these beginner exercises, you lay the groundwork for a robust memory enhancement strategy. These simple yet effective techniques provide a gentle introduction to the world of cognitive improvement, allowing you to build confidence and momentum. As you progress, you'll find yourself better equipped to tackle more advanced challenges while enjoying the benefits of a sharper, more resilient memory.

5.1 INTERMEDIATE CHALLENGES: BUILDING ON BASICS

As you become more comfortable with foundational memory exercises, it's time to introduce moderate complexity into your routine, challenging yourself just enough to stimulate growth without feeling overwhelmed. One effective way to expand on these foundational skills is through categorization tasks that require sorting information. Imagine sifting through a pile of mixed items, grouping them by color, size, or function. This exercise sharpens your ability to organize thoughts and enhances your brain's capacity for processing and retrieving information. It trains your mind to find patterns and establish connections, a crucial skill for improving memory and comprehension. Sequential memory challenges, like creating narratives or storylines, are another excellent tool. Craft a simple story where each sentence logically follows the previous one, building a coherent narrative. This task exercises your sequential processing skills, which are vital for following complex instructions or recalling detailed information.

Cognitive flexibility is a skill that allows you to adapt and thrive in various situations. To hone this ability, incorporate exercises that promote flexibility and adaptability. Consider switching tasks rapidly to test how quickly your brain can adjust. For instance, alternate between simple math problems and word puzzles, challenging your mind to shift gears efficiently. This practice enhances mental agility, making you more adept at handling unexpected changes or multitasking. Combining visual and auditory memory tasks can further improve cognitive flexibility. Listen to a short audio clip and immediately sketch a visual representation of what you heard. This exercise engages multiple senses, encouraging your brain to integrate and process information from different sources simultaneously.

Intermediate learners benefit from moderate-intensity brain workouts that require more focus and effort. Timed recall exercises are efficient for increasing speed and accuracy. Set a timer and challenge yourself to recall as many details as possible about a specific topic or event. This exercise sharpens your retrieval skills, allowing you to access stored information more quickly and accurately. Visualization drills with detailed imagery also offer significant benefits. Picture a familiar scene, such as your kitchen, and mentally walk through it, noting every detail. The more vivid your visualization, the better your brain becomes at forming and recalling complex mental images.

Tracking your progress at this intermediate level is essential for maintaining motivation and ensuring continued improvement. Begin by setting intermediate milestones for specific skills you wish to develop. These milestones provide clear targets to aim for, guiding your practice and keeping you focused. Whether improving your recall speed or mastering a new cognitive technique, setting benchmarks helps measure your success. Additionally, consider using apps designed to monitor cognitive improvements. These tools offer features like progress charts and performance metrics, providing valuable insights into your memory enhancement journey. By regularly evaluating your progress, you can identify areas for improvement and adjust your practice accordingly, ensuring that your efforts remain effective and aligned with your goals.

Interactive Element: Mid-Level Memory Challenge

Design a weekly challenge incorporating categorization tasks, cognitive flexibility exercises, and brain workouts. Track your performance each day, noting improvements or difficulties. Use this challenge to build your mental strength and adaptability gradually.

As you embrace these intermediate challenges, remember that the goal is to build on what you've already learned, moving forward with confidence and curiosity. Each exercise is a step toward greater cognitive resilience, equipping you with the tools to navigate the complexities of daily life with a sharper, more agile mind.

5.2 ADVANCED TECHNIQUES: PUSHING COGNITIVE LIMITS

Reaching the advanced stage of memory enhancement is like stepping into a world where challenges become opportunities for exploration. That is where complex memory exercises come into play, designed to push the boundaries of what your mind can achieve. Multi-step problem-solving tasks are a great start. These exercises require you to process information in stages, each step building on the previous one. Imagine tackling a complex puzzle that demands you gather clues and then piece them together methodically to reveal the bigger picture. Such tasks test your memory and strengthen your ability to integrate and recall interconnected details. Complex pattern recognition activities further elevate this challenge. Here, you engage with sequences and structures, training your brain to discern subtle patterns and relationships. It's like seeing the world in high definition, where invisible threads of logic connect everything.

Advanced visualization and recall exercises elevate your cognitive capabilities to new heights. One powerful method is creating and navigating detailed Memory Palaces. This technique involves visualizing a familiar space, like your home, and mentally placing items or information in specific locations. To recall the information, you mentally walk through the palace, retrieving each piece as you encounter it. It's a mental journey that transforms abstract data into tangible experiences, making recall more intuitive and engaging. Another exercise is memorizing long sequences or narratives. This task requires you to hold extensive information in your mind, weaving it into a coherent story. Whether it's a speech or a series of historical events, this exercise enhances your capacity for sequential recall, helping you easily manage large data sets.

Incorporating analytical thinking into your memory exercises adds depth and complexity. Logical reasoning puzzles with memory components are a perfect example. These puzzles challenge you to use deductive reasoning while retaining critical information. Imagine solving a mystery where each clue must be remembered and analyzed for significance. This dual challenge exercises memory and logic, fostering a more holistic approach to problem-solving. Strategy games that require planning and recall offer similar benefits. Games like chess or strategic card games demand foresight and the ability to remember past moves, encouraging your brain to develop an adaptable memory strategy.

Adapting to high-level challenges is crucial to maintaining progress and preventing stagnation. One way to keep your exercises fresh is by increasing complexity and adding multiple dimensions to tasks. For instance, you might combine a memory task with a time constraint or introduce a social element, like explaining your thought process to a peer. Regularly updating your exercises is also vital. As you become more adept, routines that once challenged you may lose their edge. To counteract this, continuously seek new challenges that test different aspects of your memory and cognition. This dynamic approach ensures that your brain remains engaged and responsive, ready to tackle whatever comes next.

5.3 CUSTOMIZING EXERCISES FOR PERSONAL PREFERENCES

Understanding how you learn best is a valuable tool in enhancing your memory. Each of us processes information differently, and recognizing your unique learning style can make memory exercises more effective and enjoyable. Some people are visual learners, thriving on images, diagrams, and spatial understanding. Others are auditory learners who benefit from listening and speaking. Then, some kinesthetic learners grasp concepts better through physical activity and hands-on experiences. By identifying your preferred style, you can tailor exercises to align with how you naturally think and remember. For example, incorporating colorful charts or mind maps into your study sessions can boost retention if you're a visual learner. Auditory learners might find repeating information aloud or listening to recordings helpful. Meanwhile, kinesthetic learners could benefit from physical activities that involve movement, such as tracing words in the air or using gestures to represent concepts. Adapting exercises to fit your dominant learning style can transform memory improvement from a chore into an engaging activity.

Integrating your interests and hobbies into memory exercises makes them more enjoyable and enhances their effectiveness. When you incorporate elements you are passionate about, the brain is more engaged and willing to form new connections. Consider using sports statistics for memory drills if you are a sports enthusiast. Analyzing player stats or recalling game scores can be a fun way to practice memory skills. Similarly, incorporating favorite songs or musical elements into memory tasks can be powerful. Music has a way of sticking in our minds, and tying it to information you want to remember can make recall more effortless and enjoyable. For instance, creating a playlist where each song represents a different concept or subject can help cement that information. By tapping into your interests, you create a personalized learning experience that resonates with you deeply, making memory exercises something to look forward to.

Striking a balance between structure and flexibility in your exercise routine is crucial to maintaining consistency while allowing creativity. A structured routine provides the discipline needed to practice regularly and make progress. However, too much rigidity can lead to burnout or boredom. Allow room for spontaneity by incorporating free-form exploration into your routine. That might mean dedicating a few minutes to each session to explore a new technique or exercise that intrigues you. Mixing structured exercises with these spontaneous elements keeps your routine dynamic and prevents it from becoming monotonous. The freedom to explore also encourages you to discover what works best for you, leading to a more personalized and practical approach to memory improvement.

To facilitate the customization of your memory exercises, consider using tools and resources designed to adapt to your needs. Many memory apps now offer personalization features that allow you to tailor exercises to your preferences and goals. These apps can track your progress, suggest new challenges, and adjust difficulty levels based on your performance. Journals and planners are also invaluable tools for creating tailored routines. You gain insight into the most effective strategies by recording your exercises, reflections, and achievements. This written record becomes a roadmap for your memory improvement journey, guiding you as you refine and adjust your approach. With these resources, you can adapt your exercises to your evolving needs, ensuring continued growth and engagement.

5.4 OVERCOMING PLATEAUS IN MEMORY IMPROVEMENT

As you advance in your memory enhancement efforts, you might notice a sense of stalling, where the gains you once celebrated seem to slow or even halt. This plateau in progress is typical, but recognizing its signs is crucial for moving beyond it. An indicator of stagnation can be the repetitive nature of your performance; tasks that once felt challenging now seem routine, with no noticeable improvement. Despite consistent practice, you might need to remember the same pieces of information or need help to increase your recall speed. This lack of progression can be frustrating, but it's also an opportunity to reassess and reinvigorate your approach.

Breaking through a plateau often requires a shift in strategy. Introducing novelty into your routine can be particularly effective. That does not mean abandoning your current exercises but incorporating new types that challenge your brain differently. For example, if you've been focusing on verbal memory, try exercises that tap into spatial or numerical skills. Change can reignite your brain's learning processes, creating fresh neural pathways and boosting engagement. Increasing the difficulty of familiar tasks is another powerful strategy. If you've mastered a particular memory game, add a time constraint or combine it with another challenge. That will add complexity, which forces your brain to adapt, pushing it to new heights and stimulating growth.

Revisiting your goals is an integral part of overcoming plateaus. Goals that once motivated you need reevaluation to remain relevant. Take a moment to assess whether your objectives still challenge you or if they need to become more comfortable. Setting new, ambitious milestones can provide the push to break free from stagnation. These new goals should stretch your abilities, encouraging you to explore uncharted cognitive territory. Re-evaluating initial objectives also ensures that your practice aligns with your current needs and aspirations, maintaining a sense of purpose and direction in your efforts.

Feedback plays a vital role in identifying areas for improvement and overcoming plateaus. Seeking input from peers or mentors can offer fresh perspectives on your performance. They might notice patterns or challenges you've overlooked, providing valuable insights into your strengths and areas for growth. Self-reflective practices like journaling or recording exercises can also illuminate your cognitive landscape. By regularly reviewing your experiences, you can identify trends and adjust your strategies accordingly. This process of reflection and adaptation ensures that your exercises remain effective and engaging, empowering you to push past limitations and continue growing.

Incorporating feedback into your routine enhances its effectiveness. Whether it's a suggestion from a mentor or an observation from your self-reflection, adapting your exercises based on feedback can lead to significant improvements. These adjustments involve tweaking your approach to a particular exercise, experimenting with new techniques, or revisiting foundational skills to reinforce your base. This iterative process of feedback and adaptation not only keeps your routine dynamic but also fosters a mindset of continuous learning and improvement.

Each plateau presents an opportunity to reassess and evolve, pushing your cognitive boundaries further. By embracing these strategies and maintaining an open, adaptable mindset, you can transform plateaus into stepping stones for continued memory enhancement. As you navigate these challenges, remember that progress is not always linear, and each step forward contributes to your overall growth, no matter how small. With persistence and creativity, you can overcome any plateau and unlock new levels of cognitive potential.

In this chapter, we've explored how to adapt exercises to your cognitive level, from beginner to advanced, offering strategies to push past plateaus. This progression not only enhances memory but also builds resilience and adaptability. As you continue your journey, the next chapter will delve into the role of technology in memory improvement, introducing tools and resources to support your cognitive goals further.

MAKE A DIFFERENCE WITH YOUR REVIEW

SHARE THE GIFT OF GROWTH AND WELLNESS

"The best way to find yourself is to lose yourself in the service of others."

MAHATMA GANDHI

Helping others brings joy and purpose. A simple act of kindness, done without expectation, can make the world brighter.

So, I have a small favor to ask…

Would you help someone you've never met, knowing they might benefit from you?

Who is this person? Like you, they could seek to sharpen their memory, boost their focus, or regain confidence in their mental abilities. They're looking for tools to improve their quality of life but might not know where to start.

With the **Brain Fitness Revolution**, I aim to empower individuals to strengthen their memory and enhance their lives. But to reach those who need it most, I need your help.

Here's how you can make an incredible impact:

Most people decide on a book based on its reviews. By leaving your feedback, you're helping someone discover this book—someone who could genuinely benefit from it.

Your review costs nothing but has the potential to change lives. It could help…

- …someone reignite their confidence in learning.
- …someone rediscover their mental clarity.
- …someone finds the tools to build a sharper memory.

If this book has been valuable to you, leaving a review is the quickest and most straightforward way to give back. It takes less than a minute but can create a ripple effect of positive change.

Ready to share your thoughts? Just scan the QR code below or click here:

[https://www.amazon.com/review/review-your-purchases/?asin=BOOKASIN]

If you believe in making a difference, you're already part of this mission. Thank you for being here and choosing to invest in your wellness and the well-being of others.

Warm regards,

Miles Sterling

P.S. Know someone who could benefit from this book? Sharing it with them is a priceless gift. Let's spread the power of memory improvement together.

CHAPTER SIX
USING TECHNOLOGY TO AID MEMORY IMPROVEMENT

Picture this: you're starting your morning, coffee in hand, ready to tackle the day. But as you reach for your phone, you're not just checking the weather or skimming emails. Instead, you're using a small, powerful tool to sharpen your mind. In today's digital age, technology offers many resources to enhance memory and cognitive function. With the rise of memory apps, your phone or tablet transforms into a cognitive gym, offering exercises tailored to improve mental agility and recall. This chapter explores the landscape of memory apps, guiding you to choose the right ones and integrate them seamlessly into your daily routine.

Choosing the right memory app can seem daunting, given the many options available. To find the most effective apps, consider several critical criteria. Start by reviewing user feedback and scientific backing. Apps with positive reviews and proven results are more likely to be effective. Look for customization features that tailor exercises to your specific needs and preferences. Feedback mechanisms are also crucial, helping you track progress and adjust your approach. Various exercises keep you engaged, preventing monotony and ensuring a comprehensive cognitive workout. Additionally, pay attention to the app's user interface. An intuitive, easy-to-navigate design makes you more likely to use the app consistently, enhancing its effectiveness.

Among the multitude of apps available, some have stood out for their effectiveness in enhancing memory and cognitive skills. Lumosity, for example, is a popular choice for its comprehensive approach to mental training. It offers games that target problem-solving, memory, attention, and more, all while considering lifestyle factors like mood and sleep. Peak is another standout, using evidence-based games to improve memory, language, and attention. Its structured approach encourages regular training, ensuring steady progress. Elevate focuses on skill-specific exercises, providing personalized workouts that adapt to your performance. Each app offers unique features that can contribute significantly to your memory improvement journey, providing a structured and engaging way to enhance cognitive abilities.

Incorporating memory apps into your daily life doesn't have to be overwhelming. Integrating them seamlessly is turning them into a natural part of your routine. Start by setting reminders for daily practice. A simple notification can be a gentle nudge, prompting you to engage with the app at your convenience. Consider using these apps during commute times or other downtime. Whether on the bus or waiting for an appointment, these moments can become opportunities for cognitive enhancement. By turning what might be idle time into productive sessions, you maximize both your time and mental gains. This approach ensures that memory exercises don't feel like an additional task but an integrated aspect of your day.

To truly benefit from memory apps, evaluating their impact regularly is essential. That involves tracking your progress through the app's analytics features. Many apps offer insights into your performance, highlighting areas of improvement and those needing attention. Use this data to make informed decisions about your practice, adjusting your focus to address weaknesses and build on strengths. Seeking periodic feedback from the app community can also provide valuable perspectives. Engaging with other users allows you to share experiences, tips, and encouragement, fostering community and support. This feedback loop enhances your understanding of the app's effectiveness and keeps you motivated and engaged.

Interactive Element: App Evaluation Checklist

Create a checklist to evaluate memory apps based on critical criteria: user reviews, scientific backing, customization, feedback, variety, and user interface. Use this checklist to assess and compare different apps, ensuring you choose the one that best suits your needs.

As you explore the world of memory apps, remember that these tools are just one piece of the cognitive enhancement puzzle. By choosing apps that align with your goals and integrating them thoughtfully into your routine, you unlock new possibilities for memory improvement.

6.1 VIRTUAL REALITY: IMMERSIVE MEMORY TRAINING

Imagine slipping on a headset and finding yourself in a vibrant 3D landscape surrounded by almost tangible scenes. That is the world of virtual reality (VR), a cutting-edge tool that offers immersive experiences. VR can revolutionize memory training by simulating real-life environments where you can engage in exercises that challenge your cognitive skills. Unlike traditional methods, VR places you in a dynamic setting, allowing you to interact with your surroundings in a way that stimulates multiple senses. This multi-sensory engagement enhances memory retention, helping you form stronger, more lasting connections.

VR offers unique advantages for enhancing memory. Providing immersive experiences encourages more profound engagement with content, making it easier to remember. When you navigate a digital environment, you receive instant feedback and can interact with elements in real time, which is crucial for effective learning. This interactive nature mimics real-world experiences, allowing the brain to process information more naturally. For instance, VR can recreate scenarios like navigating a busy street or exploring a historical site. Such realistic simulations enhance memory recall by embedding knowledge in familiar, contextual settings. This approach leverages the brain's natural ability to remember locations and events, making VR a powerful tool for cognitive enhancement.

Selecting the right VR program is critical to maximizing these benefits. Look for platforms like Oculus that offer learning environments specifically designed for memory training. These programs often include a variety of scenarios and tasks that target different cognitive skills. VR experiences that mimic real-world situations can be particularly effective, providing context that aids memory retention. When choosing a VR program, consider factors like content diversity, ease of use, and adaptability to your skill level. A well-designed VR experience should challenge you enough to promote growth without causing frustration. You can find the one that best suits your needs and goals by exploring different programs.

Integrating VR into your memory routines can be both exciting and rewarding. Start by scheduling weekly VR sessions, treating them as dedicated time for cognitive training. This regular practice ensures you consistently engage with the technology, maximizing its benefits. Combine VR with other memory exercises for a well-rounded approach. For example, follow a VR session with traditional exercises like puzzles or memory games. This combination reinforces learning by engaging different parts of the brain. Additionally, VR can be a motivational tool, making memory training more enjoyable and engaging. As you explore this technology, you'll likely discover new possibilities for enhancing your cognitive skills.

Interactive Element: VR Program Selection Guide

Use this guide to evaluate VR programs based on critical factors: content variety, user interface, adaptability, and feedback mechanisms. Compare different programs to find the one that aligns with your memory improvement goals.

6.2 GAMIFYING MEMORY EXERCISES FOR MOTIVATION

Imagine combining the thrill of a game with the benefits of memory exercises. That is the essence of gamification, a concept that injects game-like elements into non-game contexts to make activities more engaging and motivating. Gamification taps into our innate love for play and competition, transforming routine tasks into exciting challenges. Gamification encourages consistent participation and sustained interest by incorporating point scoring, leaderboards, and rewards. In the context of memory improvement, these elements can make exercises feel less like chores and more like engaging activities that you look forward to. This approach boosts motivation and enhances the effectiveness of memory exercises by fostering a sense of achievement and progress.

Several tools and games have successfully harnessed gamification to enhance memory exercises. Brainwell offers a suite of game-based cognitive challenges that target various skills, including memory, attention, and problem-solving. Each game is designed to be fun and stimulating, encouraging regular practice by offering new challenges and rewards. Similarly, CogniFit incorporates competitive elements, allowing you to compete against yourself or others. This competitive aspect can be particularly motivating, adding extra excitement to each session. By turning memory exercises into games, these tools bridge the gap between entertainment and education, making cognitive training a rewarding experience. Gamification transforms how we approach memory improvement, infusing it with the joy of play and the challenge of competition.

Creating personalized game-based challenges is another way to leverage gamification for memory enhancement. Start by setting up a point system for task completion. Assign points to different exercises based on their complexity or the time required to complete them. As you accumulate points, you can reward yourself with small treats or privileges, adding an element of excitement to your routine. Consider creating leaderboards with friends or family members. This social aspect introduces a friendly competition, motivating everyone to participate and improve. By personalizing the challenges, you tailor the experience to your interests and goals, ensuring it's both enjoyable and effective. This approach encourages creativity and collaboration, turning memory improvement into a shared adventure.

It's important to balance fun and effectiveness when using gamified exercises. While it's easy to get caught up in the excitement of a game, it's crucial to ensure that the activities align with your memory goals. Monitor the time spent on game activities to prevent them from becoming distractions. Set specific objectives for each session, ensuring that the chosen games target the skills you wish to improve. Keeping your goals in mind ensures that the fun and excitement translate into real cognitive gains. This balance ensures that gamification remains a tool for enhancement rather than a mere pastime, optimizing its benefits for memory improvement.

Gamification offers a dynamic approach to memory exercises, transforming them into engaging and motivating activities. By incorporating game elements into your routine, you tap into the power of play to enhance cognitive skills and memory retention. As you explore gamified tools and create personalized challenges, memory improvement becomes a more enjoyable and rewarding endeavor.

6.3 DIGITAL TOOLS FOR TRACKING MEMORY PROGRESS

Imagine having a clear snapshot of your cognitive growth before you, like a chart mapping your progress on a fitness journey. This visual representation can be incredibly motivating, offering tangible proof of your improvements in your memory skills. Digital progress tracking serves this exact purpose. It goes beyond just monitoring; it provides insight into where you excel and where you might need more focus. When you see your progress in graphs or charts, it becomes easier to recognize patterns and set realistic goals. This clarity can boost your motivation, reminding you how far you've come and the potential that lies ahead.

Selecting the right digital tools to track your memory progress is crucial. You want something that captures your activities and offers meaningful analysis. Apps like MindPal are designed with built-in progress trackers that provide detailed insights into your cognitive exercises. These apps often offer features such as activity logs, performance metrics, and visual charts to simplify data interpretation. Platforms like Google Sheets allow you to create custom tracking systems for those who prefer a more personalized approach. You can tailor these spreadsheets to include specific exercises, goals, and progress markers, making your tracking as unique as your memory journey. The key is choosing tools that align with your preferences and providing helpful feedback.

Once you have your tracking tools, the next step is to interpret the data they provide. Analyzing trends in your performance metrics can reveal a lot about your cognitive abilities. Look for patterns in your data to identify days or exercises where you perform particularly well. This reflection helps highlight your strengths, allowing you to build upon them. At the same time, be mindful of areas where you struggle. These insights are invaluable for refining your memory improvement strategies. They guide you in making informed decisions about which areas to focus on and which exercises might need adjustment. Understanding your data is like having a personal coach guiding your efforts and helping you stay on track.

With a clear understanding of your performance data, you can begin to adjust your strategies for memory improvement. Set new goals based on the insights you've gathered. If the data consistently improves one area, consider setting more challenging targets to further your abilities. Conversely, if you notice stagnation or decline, modify your routines to address these weaknesses. This might involve incorporating new exercises, increasing the frequency of certain activities, or even taking a step back to revisit foundational skills. The flexibility to adapt your approach based on data ensures that your memory training remains practical and relevant to your evolving needs.

Visual Element: Progress Tracking Template

Consider creating a template to track your memory exercises. Include columns for the date, exercise type, duration, and a notes section for reflections. This template is a tangible record of your efforts and growth, providing a clear path forward as you continue your memory journey.

6.4 INTEGRATING TECHNOLOGY WITH TRADITIONAL TECHNIQUES

In a world where digital innovations constantly emerge, there's great value in blending contemporary technology with time-tested traditional memory techniques. This hybrid approach doesn't just capitalize on the strengths of each method; it creates a dynamic memory enhancement strategy that is both flexible and robust. Combining digital exercises with physical activities can stimulate different parts of your brain, making your memory training more holistic. Imagine starting your day with a brisk walk while recalling facts or details, then using a memory app later to reinforce what you practiced. This balance ensures a comprehensive workout for your mind, engaging it in diverse ways and preventing monotony.

Successful integration of technology and traditional methods can lead to impressive results in memory improvement. For instance, consider using apps that support mnemonic devices. These digital tools can reinforce memory techniques by providing interactive exercises that adapt to your progress. You might find an app that helps you create vivid mental images or associations, complementing traditional mnemonic practices. Similarly, VR experiences paired with real-world practice can create immersive learning environments. Imagine using VR to simulate a foreign language immersion and practicing phrases with a real-life partner. This combination of virtual and tangible practice helps solidify learning, making recall more natural and intuitive.

Integrating tech-based and traditional elements into your memory improvement plan is important to develop a balanced routine. Start by scheduling tech-free days dedicated to traditional exercises. These days, focus on activities like reading, puzzles, or face-to-face conversations that challenge your memory without digital assistance. This break from screens can refresh your mind, allowing it to engage with information differently. On other days, balance screen time with offline activities. Use digital tools for structured exercises, and then apply what you've learned in real-world contexts. This approach ensures you're not overly reliant on technology, fostering a more versatile memory training regimen.

Integrating technology with traditional techniques is challenging. One common issue is managing screen fatigue, which can occur with excessive digital engagement. To combat this, set time limits for screen use and take regular breaks to rest your eyes and mind. Ensure consistent practice across both approaches by establishing a routine with diverse activities. This variety keeps your brain engaged and prevents burnout, ensuring that memory training remains effective and enjoyable. It's also important to remain flexible and willing to adjust your strategy as needed, recognizing that what works best may change over time.

A hybrid approach to memory improvement combines the best of both worlds. Integrating technology and traditional methods creates a dynamic and effective memory training strategy. This balance enhances your cognitive abilities and ensures that memory exercises remain engaging and sustainable.

CHAPTER SEVEN
ADDRESSING COMMON MEMORY IMPROVEMENT BARRIERS

Imagine standing in a vast library where the books are all the experiences and knowledge you've gathered over the years. Now imagine some of those books slowly slipping off the shelves without warning. This unsettling image captures the fear many experience when they first notice signs of cognitive decline. It's a fear steeped in misconceptions, often exacerbated by the belief that aging will eventually lead to memory loss. However, understanding cognitive decline involves separating myth from reality.

Contrary to popular belief, not all memory lapses signal a deteriorating mind. Many older adults maintain a sharp memory well into their later years, thanks to cognitive resilience and active mental engagement. Scientific studies consistently show that while some cognitive changes are natural with age, they don't necessarily lead to significant memory loss or dementia.

Recognizing early signs of cognitive decline is crucial in addressing these fears. It's important to differentiate between normal memory lapses and those warranting professional attention. Forgetting the name of an acquaintance or occasionally misplacing items can be normal, especially during busy periods. However, struggling to follow familiar routes or frequently forgetting conversations might indicate more serious concerns. Understanding these differences can guide you in seeking appropriate help if needed. A professional evaluation can provide clarity, offering reassurance or early intervention. Maintaining awareness without letting fear dictate your perception of memory changes is important.

Taking proactive steps can significantly mitigate the risk of cognitive decline. Engaging in regular mental exercises, such as puzzles, crosswords, or learning a new language, can keep your brain active and healthy. These activities stimulate neural connections and promote cognitive resilience, as physical exercise strengthens muscles. A healthy lifestyle, rich in balanced nutrition, also supports brain function. Foods high in omega-3 fatty acids, antioxidants, and other brain-boosting nutrients fuel cognitive processes. Staying hydrated and maintaining a diet abundant in fruits, vegetables, and whole grains can foster a brain-friendly environment, helping to preserve memory over time.

Building cognitive reserve is another strategy to buffer against decline. This concept refers to the brain's ability to improvise and find alternative ways of completing tasks. It acts as a safety net, allowing the brain to adapt to changes and challenges. Engaging in activities that challenge and expand your cognitive abilities contributes to this reserve. Learning new skills, whether a musical instrument, a craft, or even a new sport, can strengthen cognitive pathways and increase brain resilience. Social engagement, such as participating in community groups or clubs, also plays a role. These activities encourage mental stimulation and emotional support, contributing to a robust cognitive reserve.

Interactive Element: Early Signs Reflection Exercise

Reflect on your daily life and identify any memory lapses you've experienced recently. Consider whether these are typical forgetfulness or if they need further attention. This exercise aims to help you discern between normal aging and potential cognitive decline, providing clarity and confidence in understanding your memory health.

Addressing these concerns and implementing proactive measures can reduce the fear associated with cognitive decline. Understanding the myths and realities, recognizing early signs, and building mental resilience can empower you to maintain your cognitive health.

7.1 MANAGING TIME: INCORPORATING EXERCISES INTO BUSY SCHEDULES

Life can feel like a never-ending race, with each day packed with commitments and responsibilities. It's easy to pay attention to the importance of memory exercises when juggling work, family, and social obligations. However, fitting these exercises into your busy schedule is possible and can significantly enhance your mental agility. Prioritizing tasks with a focus on cognitive health is a crucial first step. Consider what tasks require immediate attention and which can be delegated or postponed. This approach frees up time and mental space, allowing you to dedicate moments to memory improvement. Time-blocking is another effective strategy. By setting aside specific blocks of time for memory exercises, you create a routine that respects your schedule and cognitive needs. These blocks don't have to be long; even 10 to 15 minutes of focused practice can yield substantial benefits.

Finding hidden opportunities for memory exercises throughout your day can transform seemingly mundane moments into valuable cognitive training sessions. Commute times, for instance, offer a unique chance to engage in audio memory exercises. Listening to podcasts or audiobooks that challenge your recall abilities can turn your daily travels into a mental workout. Similarly, lunch breaks provide a brief respite from work that you can use for short, engaging memory tasks. Whether it's a quick word association game or a few minutes of meditation to clear your mind, these activities can refresh and refocus your brain for the afternoon ahead. Identifying these pockets of time makes memory exercises more manageable and integrates them seamlessly into your daily life.

Flexibility is key in choosing memory improvement activities that suit your hectic lifestyle. Quick recall challenges, like memorizing a list of words or numbers in a minute, require minimal time but can sharpen your memory skills significantly. Smartphone apps designed for cognitive training offer another flexible option. These apps often feature short, engaging exercises you can complete while waiting in line or during a coffee break. They adapt to your schedule, providing on-the-go opportunities to enhance your memory without needing a formal setting or extensive preparation. By embracing flexible exercises, you ensure that memory improvement remains a consistent part of your life, regardless of how busy your days become.

Forming consistent habits is vital in regular practice and reaping the benefits of memory exercises. Daily reminders help establish these habits, prompting you to engage in memory activities even on the busiest days. Over time, these reminders become ingrained in your routine, making memory practice as habitual as brushing your teeth. Creating a routine incorporating cognitive activities encourages regular engagement and helps prevent memory exercises from becoming an afterthought. The key is consistency, whether a morning brain teaser or an evening reflection exercise. As these practices become routine, they reinforce your memory skills, leading to gradual and sustainable improvement.

7.2 DEALING WITH DISCOURAGEMENT: HOW TO STAY MOTIVATED

When you first set out to improve your memory, there's an initial burst of enthusiasm. You envision a future where recalling names and details is second nature. Yet, as days turn into weeks, this bright optimism can dim. One common source of discouragement is the need for immediate results. It's natural to want quick wins, but memory improvement is often gradual. This delay can lead to frustration, causing you to doubt the effectiveness of your efforts. Another pitfall is the tendency to compare yourself to others. Perhaps you have a friend who seems to breeze through memory exercises while you're struggling to see progress. This comparison can sap your motivation, leaving you feeling inadequate. It's crucial to remember that everyone's cognitive journey is unique; progress varies from person to person based on numerous factors, including past experiences and current practices.

Maintaining motivation requires strategies that keep you engaged and hopeful. Celebrating small victories is a powerful tool in this regard. Every step forward, no matter how minor, is a testament to your dedication. Did you remember your grocery list without looking? That's a win. Acknowledging these successes fosters a sense of accomplishment and boosts your confidence. Setting realistic and achievable goals is also vital. Lofty goals can be daunting, but breaking them into manageable tasks makes them more approachable. Instead of aiming to memorize a lengthy poem in one go, start with a single stanza. This gradual approach creates a series of attainable targets, each bringing you closer to your ultimate objective. These smaller victories accumulate, reinforcing your commitment and proving that progress is possible.

Positive reinforcement can further enhance your motivation. Reward systems are effective for sustaining momentum. Consider setting milestones and treating yourself upon reaching them. Rewards don't have to be extravagant; a favorite snack or a relaxing bath can motivate you to keep going. Visualization is another powerful tool, allowing you to picture the long-term benefits of your efforts. Imagine how improved memory will enhance your life, from better work performance to richer social interactions. This mental image can be a beacon, guiding you through the challenges and reminding you of your ultimate goal. The promise of these benefits can inspire perseverance, even when the road seems long.

Setbacks are inevitable, but they don't have to derail your efforts. Instead of viewing them as failures, see them as opportunities for growth. Every challenge encountered is a chance to learn more about yourself and your methods. Reflecting on these moments can reveal areas for improvement, helping you adjust your strategies effectively. A particular exercise needs to yield the desired results. Use this insight to explore alternative methods that might suit you better. The willingness to adapt is crucial. Flexibility allows you to pivot when needed, ensuring your progress continues despite obstacles. Reframing setbacks in this way transforms potential roadblocks into stepping stones, paving the way for greater achievements. Embracing this mindset fosters resilience and encourages a proactive approach to memory improvement.

Interactive Element: Motivation Reflection Section

Take a few moments to reflect on your own memory improvement journey. Identify a recent victory, no matter how small. How did it make you feel, and how can you build on it? Consider a setback you've encountered. What did it teach you, and how might you adjust your approach? Jot down your reflections in a journal. This exercise can provide clarity and reinforce your commitment to sustained progress.

7.3 FINDING SUPPORT: BUILDING A MEMORY IMPROVEMENT COMMUNITY

Imagine sitting in a room with people who fully understand what you're going through. There's something deeply comforting about knowing you're not alone in your struggles with memory. Engaging with a supportive community offers numerous benefits, from sharing experiences to gaining new insights. You can learn from others who have faced similar challenges when you're part of a community. You might discover new techniques or strategies that you still need to consider. Besides practical advice, the emotional support from peers who empathize with your situation can be invaluable. They can offer encouragement on tough days and celebrate with you on better ones.

Forming or joining a memory improvement group can provide structure and support. Local community groups often focus on cognitive health, organizing regular meetings or workshops where members can share their experiences and learn from one another. Check with your community center or local library for information on such groups. If in-person meetings aren't feasible, online forums and social media groups offer virtual support. These platforms connect you with others regardless of location, allowing for a diverse exchange of ideas and encouragement. Engaging in these communities can make memory improvement less daunting and more collaborative.

Collaborative learning opportunities within these communities can enhance the experience further. Group memory games or challenges are fun and a great way to practice cognitive skills in a supportive environment. These activities can foster a sense of camaraderie, making memory exercises feel less like a solitary task. Peer-led workshops and skill-sharing sessions can also be incredibly beneficial. Members can share their expertise or experiences, leading sessions on memory techniques or lifestyle adjustments supporting cognitive health. This shared learning can inspire new approaches and deepen your understanding of memory improvement.

Several resources and platforms can help find or establish a supportive network. Websites dedicated to cognitive health often list local initiatives and events. They can be a good starting point for locating community activities. Apps designed for memory improvement also have features that connect users with others, facilitating the creation of virtual support networks. For those looking to start their own group, community bulletin boards and online platforms like Meetup can be effective tools for gathering interested individuals. Building or joining a community dedicated to memory improvement enhances your journey and provides a sense of belonging and shared purpose.

ADDRESSING COMMON MEMORY IMPROVEMENT BARRIERS 93

Visual Element: Community Support Checklist

Create a checklist to evaluate potential memory support groups based on location, meeting frequency, and focus areas. This tool can help you identify which groups align best with your needs and preferences, guiding your decision on where to seek support.

7.4 COMMUNICATING YOUR MEMORY NEEDS TO FAMILY AND FRIENDS

Navigating the maze of memory challenges can feel overwhelming, especially when articulating your needs to those closest to you. It's crucial to communicate effectively, ensuring your loved ones understand what you're experiencing. Begin by expressing your feelings and needs clearly. Using "I" statements can be a powerful tool in this context. For instance, saying, "I feel frustrated when I can't remember appointments," helps convey your experience without placing blame. It's a way to open a dialogue without creating defensiveness. Sharing specific examples of your memory difficulties can further illuminate your situation. You frequently need to remember the names of people you've just met or struggle to recall recent conversations. Providing concrete instances gives your family a clearer picture of your daily challenges.

Educating your family and friends about memory issues fosters understanding and empathy. While you might be keenly aware of the nuances of your memory challenges, they might not grasp the extent or nature of your struggles. Providing them with reading materials on cognitive health can be enlightening. These resources can demystify memory issues, debunk myths, and offer insight into what you're facing. Inviting your loved ones to participate in learning sessions or workshops on memory can also be beneficial.

These events educate and provide a shared experience, helping them see the world from your perspective. Their involvement can deepen their understanding and reinforce the importance of their support in your journey.

Requesting support from your family and friends is crucial in your memory improvement efforts. Don't hesitate to ask for help setting up reminders or cues around the house. Whether it's sticky notes with important dates or electronic reminders for daily tasks, these aids can make a significant difference. Involving your family in memory exercises or activities can also be beneficial. Engaging in memory games or discussing techniques over a meal boosts your cognitive skills and strengthens familial bonds. Their participation can transform memory exercises from solitary tasks into communal activities, fostering a sense of teamwork and shared purpose.

The environment at home plays a significant role in your memory improvement journey. A supportive home environment can enhance your cognitive efforts, making them more effective and enjoyable. Encouraging open dialogue about cognitive health is essential. Regular conversations about memory, challenges, and progress can normalize the topic, reducing stigma or embarrassment. Establishing family routines that prioritize mental well-being can further support your memory goals. That might involve setting aside time for shared relaxation activities, like reading or meditating together. Such routines promote mental wellness and create a nurturing atmosphere that supports memory enhancement.

Effective communication of memory needs can create a bridge of understanding with your loved ones. This connection can transform your memory improvement efforts from a solitary endeavor into a collaborative journey enriched by the support and empathy of those closest to you. As you continue to navigate the complexities of memory improvement, remember that the support of family and friends can be a powerful ally, offering encouragement and solace along the way.

This chapter explored the importance of communicating memory needs to loved ones, fostering understanding, and building a supportive environment. As we progress, we'll delve into holistic approaches to cognitive health, exploring how lifestyle choices influence memory and overall well-being.

CHAPTER EIGHT
HOLISTIC APPROACHES TO COGNITIVE HEALTH

Imagine your brain as the conductor of an intricate orchestra, where each section represents a different aspect of your health, working in harmony to produce the symphony of your life. Physical health, nutrition, and cardiovascular wellness each play a role in this concert, impacting your body and memory. It might seem surprising, but the movement of your body and the food you eat can influence how well you remember a friend's phone number, your grocery list, or even the details of your favorite novel.

8.1 THE CONNECTION BETWEEN PHYSICAL HEALTH AND MEMORY

Regular physical exercise is like a power-up for your brain. Engaging in aerobic activities, such as brisk walking or cycling, toning your muscles and boosting your brain volume. This increase in volume, particularly in areas related to memory and learning, suggests a healthier, more robust brain. Aerobic exercises improve blood flow, ensuring your brain receives the nutrients and oxygen needed to function optimally. Strength training, too, plays a vital role by increasing neural growth factors, which are proteins that support the survival of neurons and the growth of new ones. These exercises create a fertile environment for neuroplasticity, the brain's ability to adapt and grow, essential for memory enhancement (SOURCE 1).

A balanced diet is another cornerstone of cognitive performance. Antioxidants in foods like berries and dark chocolate help reduce oxidative stress, a process that can damage cells and lead to cognitive decline. These powerful compounds act as scavengers, neutralizing harmful molecules that threaten brain health. Meanwhile, healthy fats, such as those in avocados and nuts, are crucial for maintaining the integrity of brain cell membranes. These fats ensure that cells communicate effectively, supporting processes like memory and learning. Together, antioxidants and healthy fats create a dietary foundation that supports and protects your cognitive abilities.

Your cardiovascular health also plays a significant role in memory function. The heart and brain are intricately linked, with blood flow as a vital connector. When your cardiovascular system is healthy, it efficiently delivers oxygen-rich blood to your brain, supporting cognitive tasks and memory retention. Conversely, hypertension, or high blood pressure, poses a risk to mental health by damaging blood vessels and reducing blood flow to the brain. This decrease can impair memory and increase the risk of cognitive decline. Maintaining cardiovascular health through regular physical activity and a heart-healthy diet bolsters your brain's resilience and functionality.

Incorporating physical health practices into your daily routine can be manageable. Start with setting achievable fitness goals, a 15-minute walk daily, or a short strength-training session twice a week. These small steps can lead to significant improvements in both physical and cognitive health. Consider combining physical activity with cognitive tasks. Walking meetings, for example, can stimulate both your body and mind, turning a simple stroll into an opportunity for mental engagement. By weaving these practices into your routine, you create an environment that supports memory and overall well-being.

Interactive Element: Fitness and Memory Journal Prompt

Reflect on your current physical activity and dietary habits. Identify one small change you can make in each area to support your brain health. Write down your plan and track your progress over the next month. Consider noting any changes in your memory or cognitive function as you incorporate these new habits.

Physical health and memory are profoundly interconnected. By nurturing your body through exercise, a balanced diet, and cardiovascular care, you lay the groundwork for a sharper, more resilient mind. These elements work together, creating a symphony that harmonizes your cognitive health and overall well-being.

8.2 STRESS MANAGEMENT TECHNIQUES FOR BETTER MEMORY

Stress, a persistent companion in modern life, can profoundly impact your memory and cognitive function. When you're stressed, your body releases cortisol, a hormone that, while helpful in short bursts, can be detrimental over time. Imagine cortisol as a flood that, in controlled doses, irrigates your brain, helping you focus and respond to immediate challenges. However, when stress lingers, cortisol becomes a relentless torrent, eroding the hippocampus, the brain's memory center. This erosion can lead to hippocampal atrophy, where the structure shrinks, compromising its ability to form and recall memories. Chronic stress acts like a slow poison, altering your brain's architecture and making it harder to hold on to new information. That is why you might struggle to remember names or important tasks when life's pressures mount.

Addressing stress requires practical approaches that provide relief and foster long-term resilience. One immediate technique is deep breathing, a simple yet powerful tool to calm your mind. Picture yourself in a moment of tension; a few deep, intentional breaths can slow your heart rate and create a sense of peace. This exercise activates the parasympathetic nervous system, which counters the stress response and promotes relaxation. For ongoing stress management, progressive muscle relaxation can be a game-changer. This method involves tensing and relaxing each muscle group, releasing built-up tension and promoting tranquility. Regular practice teaches your body and mind to release stress, paving the way for a clearer, more focused mind.

Mindfulness and meditation offer pathways to more profound stress reduction and memory enhancement. Guided meditation apps can serve as your personal coach, walking you through exercises designed to reduce stress and improve cognitive function. These apps often include sessions focused on calming the mind and cultivating awareness, which can be particularly beneficial in managing stress. Mindful breathing exercises, where you focus solely on each inhale and exhale, reinforce this calmness. This practice anchors you in the present moment, reducing the mental chatter that often accompanies stress. Over time, incorporating mindfulness into your daily routine can transform how you respond to life's pressures, enhancing memory and overall well-being.

Building resilience to stress is about creating a buffer that shields you from life's inevitable storms. Cognitive-behavioral strategies offer practical ways to reframe negative thoughts and develop a more balanced perspective. You can reduce their impact on your mood and memory by identifying and challenging unhelpful thought patterns. Additionally, developing a support network provides a crucial foundation for emotional strength. Surrounding yourself with people who understand and support you can significantly affect how you handle stress. Whether it's friends, family, or a support group, these connections offer a safe space to share your experiences and gain perspective.

Interactive Element: Stress Reflection Section

Take a quiet moment to reflect on what causes stress and how it affects your memory. Write down any patterns you notice and consider which stress management techniques might be most helpful for you to explore. This exercise can be a starting point for developing a more effective stress management strategy.

8.3 SLEEP AND ITS ROLE IN MEMORY CONSOLIDATION

Sleep is not merely a time for rest; it's a dynamic period where your brain engages in vital processes that bolster memory and learning. Your brain processes emotional memories during sleep, particularly in rapid eye movement (REM). Imagine your mind sifting through the day's experiences, deciding which memories to keep and which to let go. This sorting process strengthens emotional recollections and helps you handle future experiences with greater insight. Slow-wave sleep, called deep sleep, plays a different yet equally crucial role. During this phase, your brain consolidates declarative memories, like facts and concepts. It transfers information from short-term to long-term storage, ensuring that what you've learned firmly takes root. This stage is vital for solidifying knowledge, making it easier to recall information when needed.

Sleep disorders can significantly disrupt these processes, leading to cognitive decline. Insomnia, characterized by difficulty falling or staying asleep, deprives your brain of the deep rest it requires. Lack of sleep can lead to symptoms like forgetfulness, difficulty concentrating, and mood swings, affecting your daily life and mental clarity. Sleep apnea, another common disorder, involves repeated interruptions in breathing during sleep, which can seriously impact your sleep quality. Disruptions like these can prevent you from reaching the deeper stages of sleep, which are essential for memory consolidation. Addressing these issues is key to improving cognitive health. Identifying sleep-related problems requires paying attention to your body's signals. If you often feel tired despite a full night's sleep, it might be time to consult a healthcare professional. They can offer solutions ranging from lifestyle changes to medical treatments that restore restful sleep and enhance cognitive function.

To improve sleep hygiene, start by establishing a sleep routine. Going to sleep and waking up at the same time daily will regulate the internal clock in your body. This makes it easier to fall asleep and wake up refreshed. Create a sleep-friendly environment by reducing electronic distractions. The blue light the screens emanate will interfere with melatonin production, the hormone regulating sleep. Consider setting a digital curfew and turning off devices at least an hour before bedtime. Instead, read a book or warm bath to calm your body. These practices signal your brain that it's time to relax and wind down, promoting relaxation and better sleep quality. Additionally, maintain a comfortable sleep environment by keeping your bedroom cool, dark, and quiet. A supportive mattress and pillows that significantly affect sleep quality may be a good investment.

When used wisely, napping can be a valuable tool for enhancing memory and cognitive function. Short naps, around 10 to 20 minutes, can provide a quick refresh without inducing grogginess. These "power naps" boost alertness and improve mood, making them an excellent option for a midday energy boost. For those with more time, a 60-minute nap can enhance memory by allowing you to enter the deeper stages of sleep. However, be cautious with longer naps, which may interfere with nighttime sleep. Incorporating naps into your routine involves finding the right balance. Consider scheduling a short nap when your energy wanes, ideally in the early afternoon. This timing helps avoid disrupting your nighttime sleep. Remember, the goal is to complement, not replace, your regular sleep, ensuring that both nighttime rest and daytime naps contribute to a well-rested mind.

Sleep's role in memory consolidation underscores the importance of prioritizing rest in daily routine. Understanding and addressing sleep challenges can enhance cognitive function and improve quality of life.

8.4 THE IMPACT OF SOCIAL INTERACTION ON COGNITIVE FUNCTION

Imagine your brain as a complex network of pathways, much like a bustling city. Each interaction you have, every conversation and social event, acts as a car traveling these roads, keeping them busy and well-maintained. Social engagement plays an integral role in maintaining cognitive health and vitality. When you engage in social activities, whether a casual chat with a neighbor or a community club meeting, you stimulate mental processes that keep your mind nimble and alert. These interactions challenge your brain to process information, respond to cues, and recall memories, all of which contribute to building cognitive resilience. A robust social network acts as a safety net, providing emotional support and mental stimulation that helps fortify your brain against the wear and tear of time.

Loneliness, however, can harm your cognitive function, like neglecting maintenance on those city roads. When you're isolated, your brain misses the stimulation and challenge social interactions provide. The absence of these interactions can lead to a decline in mental sharpness and memory. Loneliness affects your mental state and can also have physiological effects, leading to increased stress and a weakened immune system. Combined factors can accelerate cognitive decline, so fostering meaningful connections is crucial. Building these connections can be manageable. Make a significant difference with simple acts like joining a book club or scheduling regular coffee dates with friends. Engaging with others creates opportunities for your brain to stay active and engaged.

Community involvement offers a powerful boost to your cognitive health. Participating in community activities or volunteering provides a sense of purpose and fosters connections with like-minded individuals. These activities present opportunities for life-long learning as you interact with people from diverse backgrounds and experiences. Volunteering, in particular, strengthens social bonds as you work alongside others toward a common goal. This sense of belonging and contribution enhances your mood and sharpens your cognitive abilities. Engaging with your community allows you to give and receive support, creating a social fabric that enriches your life and keeps your mind sharp.

Developing social skills is closely linked to memory improvement. Role-playing activities can enhance your social skills, providing a safe space to practice communication and empathy. By putting yourself in different scenarios, you exercise your ability to interpret social cues and respond appropriately, stimulating your brain. Group discussions also offer valuable opportunities to improve recall and communication. When you participate in a debate, your brain is tasked with remembering details, forming coherent thoughts, and conveying them effectively. This exercise strengthens neural connections related to memory and communication skills, contributing to a more agile mind.

Interactive Element: Social Engagement Reflection Exercise

Reflect on your current level of social engagement. Consider the activities you participate in and the connections you maintain. Write down one or two new social activities you might try to enhance your cognitive function. That could be anything from joining a local club to volunteering at a community event. Note how these activities could challenge your brain and enrich your life.

8.5 CREATING A BALANCED LIFESTYLE FOR OPTIMAL MEMORY HEALTH

In the hustle and bustle of everyday life, finding balance can feel like a juggling act. Yet, this very balance lays the foundation for optimal cognitive health. It's not just about one aspect of life but about integrating physical, mental, and social activities into a harmonious whole. When you engage in various activities, your brain benefits from the diverse stimuli, each encouraging different neural pathways to develop and strengthen. This variety keeps your mind agile, ready to adapt to new challenges, and more robust in the face of stress. Prioritizing self-care is crucial, too. It's about taking the time for yourself through mindfulness practices that ground you or simply finding moments to breathe deeply and reflect. This self-care acts as a buffer against the demands of daily life, reducing stress and enhancing your ability to focus and remember.

Time management plays a crucial role in maintaining this balance. You create a structure that supports mental well-being by managing your time effectively. Scheduling regular breaks throughout your day provides mental rejuvenation, allowing you to return to tasks with renewed focus and clarity. These breaks act as mini-resets, helping to prevent burnout and maintain productivity. Allocating time for hobbies and relaxation is equally important. Engaging in activities you love brings joy and stimulates different areas of your brain, promoting overall cognitive health. Whether painting, playing an instrument, or simply walking in nature, these leisure moments contribute to a well-rounded, satisfying life.

Mental health, often overlooked, is an integral part of living a balanced lifestyle. Recognizing signs of mental fatigue and burnout is essential. Symptoms might include irritability, forgetfulness, or a constant feeling overwhelmed. When these signs appear, it's crucial to acknowledge them and take proactive steps to address them. Seeking professional help through therapy or counseling can provide valuable support and guidance. It's a step towards understanding and managing mental health challenges, supporting memory and cognitive function. Remember, mental health is as important as physical health; nurturing it can significantly improve your quality of life.

Cultivating positive habits paves the way for enhanced cognitive health and overall well-being. Developing a routine that supports healthy sleep, nutrition, and exercise creates a stable foundation for your day. A regular sleep schedule ensures your brain gets the rest it needs to function optimally. A balanced diet fuels your brain, providing the nutrients necessary for cognitive processes. Regular exercise keeps your body and mind fit, enhancing your ability to focus and remember. Practicing gratitude and positive thinking can also bolster mental resilience. Focusing on the positives in life creates a more adaptable mindset to challenges, reducing stress and promoting a sense of well-being. These habits, while simple, profoundly impact your cognitive health and can significantly improve memory and focus.

Creating a balanced lifestyle requires effort and awareness, but the rewards are worth it. Integrating diverse activities, managing your time wisely, maintaining mental health, and cultivating positive habits fosters an environment where your mind can thrive. This holistic approach supports memory and enhances your overall quality of life. As you continue this journey of cognitive enhancement, remember that each step you take contributes to a healthier, more vibrant mind. The next chapter will explore real-life success stories, showcasing how these strategies have transformed lives and inspired change.

CHAPTER NINE
REAL-LIFE SUCCESS STORIES AND TESTIMONIALS

Picture this: a bustling office, phones ringing, papers shuffling, and amidst the chaos, a professional stands confidently, recalling every detail of a complex presentation without a single note. That isn't a scene from a movie but a real-life success story of memory improvement in action. Memory is not just about recalling facts; it's about enriching your life, improving your relationships, and opening doors to new opportunities. This chapter unfolds the stories of individuals who have transformed their lives by enhancing their memory, proving that change is possible at any age and stage.

Meet Sarah, a senior citizen who once struggled with social interactions due to forgetfulness. Invitations dwindled as she hesitated to join conversations, fearing she might need to remember names or critical details. But Sarah decided to take charge. She began a program of consistent cognitive training, incorporating simple daily exercises like word puzzles and memory games. Over time, her efforts paid off. She regained her confidence, started attending social gatherings, and even became a regular member of a community book club. The transformation was profound; her memory improvement enriched her social life, bringing joy and fulfillment she hadn't felt in years.

Then there's Tom, a busy marketing executive juggling deadlines and demanding clients. Tom realized his career was suffering because he often needed to remember essential meeting points and client preferences. Determined to improve, he explored memory enhancement techniques and discovered the Memory Palace method. Tom delivered presentations with newfound confidence and clarity by associating key presentation points with familiar locations in his home. His improved recall and communication skills not only bolstered his performance at work but also led to a promotion and increased responsibilities. Memory improvement became the key to unlocking Tom's potential, paving the way for career advancement and personal growth.

Memory enhancement also brings unexpected benefits, transforming professional and personal lives. For many, improved memory leads to stronger relationships. Remembering birthdays, anniversaries, and meaningful moments strengthens bonds, showing loved ones they are valued and cherished. Improved recall fosters better communication, reducing misunderstandings and deepening connections. Engaging fully in conversations and recalling past discussions and shared experiences enhances relationships, creating a foundation of trust and intimacy. Memory, thus, becomes more than just a tool for information; it becomes a bridge connecting hearts and minds.

The techniques that fueled these transformations are diverse and adaptable, allowing individuals to tailor them to their needs. Alongside the Memory Palace, techniques like mindfulness play a crucial role. Incorporating mindfulness into daily routines helps individuals maintain focus and clarity. Simple practices such as mindful breathing or meditation foster a calm mind, reducing the noise of distractions and enhancing memory. These techniques are accessible and practical, making them suitable for anyone seeking to improve their cognitive abilities. By integrating these methods into daily life, individuals find enhanced memory and a renewed sense of purpose and well-being.

Personal milestones mark the memory improvement journey, providing tangible evidence of growth and achievement. Completing a challenging educational course or remembering essential dates continually are milestones worth celebrating. Each represents a victory over forgetfulness, a testament to dedication and hard work. These milestones motivate and encourage continued effort and exploration of new memory techniques. They remind individuals that memory improvement is a journey marked by perseverance and progress, where each step forward is a step toward a more fulfilling life.

Interactive Element: Reflection Exercise

Reflect on your memory journey. Identify a milestone you hope to achieve—perhaps remembering a loved one's birthday without a reminder or learning a new skill. Jot down the steps to reach this goal, noting any techniques you plan to use. This reflection can serve as a guide, helping you visualize your path to memory improvement.

9.1 LESSONS LEARNED: WHAT WORKED FOR OTHERS

One element stands out across countless stories of memory improvement: consistency in practice. This simple yet profound principle underpins many success stories. Even in small amounts, regular training gradually builds more robust memory pathways. Imagine you're planting a garden. Each day, you water it, tending it with care, and eventually, you see the fruits of your labor. Memory works in much the same way. Consistency transforms the abstract into the attainable, anchoring new techniques into everyday life. Many who have succeeded in improving their memory found that setting achievable, incremental goals made all the difference. It's not about memorizing an entire book overnight but perhaps starting with a single page. This approach helps keep motivation high, as each small victory paves the path to more significant accomplishments.

Adapting memory techniques to fit personal lifestyles is another common thread among successful individuals. Life is busy, and only some have the luxury of dedicating daily hours to memory exercises. Those who have succeeded often tailored techniques to mesh with their unique schedules. For some, this meant using quiet moments during commutes to practice mental imagery or using an app with spaced repetition exercises during lunch breaks. Others found ways to incorporate their hobbies into their memory practice, which made the process more engaging. A music lover might associate notes with visual imagery, while a cooking enthusiast might memorize recipes by creating vivid mental pictures of each ingredient. Personalizing exercises enhances effectiveness and makes the process enjoyable, blending seamlessly into one's lifestyle.

Initial challenges are inevitable but can be overcome with the right mindset. Skepticism is often a barrier, especially for those new to memory techniques. Many begin with doubt, still determining if these methods will yield actual results. It's essential to remain open-minded and willing to experiment. Consider it a scientific endeavor where trial and error lead to discovery. Those who push past initial skepticism often find themselves pleasantly surprised by their progress. Embracing new techniques, even unconventional, can open doors to unexpected improvements. For example, someone might initially doubt the effectiveness of mnemonic devices, only to find them incredibly helpful in memorizing complex information once they give them a fair trial.

Patience and persistence are the unsung heroes in the journey of memory improvement. Real change doesn't happen overnight; it requires time and dedication. Celebrating small victories is crucial. Each step forward, no matter how minor, deserves recognition. These moments of progress are affirmations of your effort and commitment. They serve as reminders that you are moving in the right direction. Persistence means continuing to practice, even on days when it feels challenging. It involves pushing through plateaus, adapting techniques, and focusing on your goals. With patience, memory improvement becomes less about immediate results and more about gradual, lasting change. The journey is long, but the rewards—greater confidence, improved relationships, and enhanced cognitive abilities—are worth the effort.

9.2 OVERCOMING SETBACKS: STORIES OF PERSISTENCE

In the memory improvement journey, setbacks are as common as the successes they precede. One prevalent challenge many face is the temporary regression in memory performance. Imagine having made strides in recalling names or details, only to experience a week where everything seems to slip through the cracks. Such regressions can be disheartening, shaking the confidence of even the most diligent. Then there are the external stressors—those unexpected events that disrupt focus and concentration. A stressful week at work or a personal crisis can cloud the mind, making it difficult to concentrate on memory exercises or daily tasks. These challenges can make the path to improved memory feel like a winding road with more obstacles than straightaways.

Yet, the stories of those who have persisted offer valuable lessons in resilience. One strategy many have found effective is seeking support from mentors or peers. Having someone to share experiences with during tough times can provide much-needed encouragement. Mentors can offer advice from their own experiences, helping to identify what might be derailing progress and suggesting ways to get back on track. Meanwhile, peers on a similar path can empathize and provide motivation, creating an incredibly uplifting camaraderie. Another approach is revisiting and adjusting goals. When faced with a setback, sometimes our goals need tweaking to remain relevant and achievable. This adjustment helps maintain motivation and ensures that efforts align with personal aspirations.

Learning from failure is another cornerstone of persistence. Many who face initial failures discover these moments rich with learning opportunities. Consider the story of a teacher who initially struggled with memory techniques, feeling overwhelmed by the sheer volume of information to be retained. Instead of giving up, they analyzed their approach, identifying that their methods were too rigid. This realization led them to explore more flexible memory aids. Eventually, they improved their memory significantly and developed new teaching methods to help students with similar challenges. By viewing failures as stepping stones, individuals can transform setbacks into valuable insights, paving the way for future success.

Celebrating resilience and determination is essential. It's about acknowledging the grit and resolve that keeps individuals moving forward despite obstacles. There are countless stories of those who, through sheer determination, achieved significant gains. Take, for instance, a young artist who used memory techniques to remember complex color patterns and compositions. Initially, they faced setbacks, forgetting key elements and feeling frustrated. However, their persistence paid off, and over time, they honed their skills to a degree where their work began to receive critical acclaim. The determination to push through difficulties, to adjust strategies, and to keep striving, even when progress seemed elusive, led to a transformation that was as personal as it was professional.

Textual Element: Reflection Section

Reflect on a personal setback you have faced in your memory improvement efforts. Identify the factors contributing to the challenge and consider how you might approach it differently next time. Write down these reflections, focusing on strategies to turn potential failures into learning opportunities.

9.3 THE POWER OF COMMUNITY IN MEMORY IMPROVEMENT

Imagine a bustling coffee shop, the air filled with chatter and laughter. In one corner, a group of individuals gathers for coffee to support each other in their quest to enhance memory. This scene captures the essence of community in memory improvement. Support networks, whether in-person or online, are pivotal in facilitating progress. They provide a safe space for sharing experiences, exchanging tips, and offering encouragement. Participants often form study groups, meeting regularly to review techniques, practice exercises, and hold each other accountable. That shared learning experience fosters a sense of belonging, helping each participant feel connected and understood.

Online support forums offer another layer of community. These forums are a haven for those seeking advice or simply a listening ear from people who understand their challenges. The digital age has made it easier than ever to connect with like-minded individuals, regardless of location. Members can share stories of triumphs and setbacks through these platforms, receive feedback, and find motivation. The camaraderie built within these spaces can be immensely empowering. It's a reminder that you are not alone in your journey and that others are navigating similar paths, ready to celebrate your successes and support you through challenges.

Engaging in group activities brings another dimension to memory improvement. Group memory games, for instance, are fun and foster a spirit of healthy competition. These games challenge participants to think quickly and recall information under pressure, honing their memory skills in a dynamic setting. Collaborative workshops, on the other hand, create opportunities for skill-sharing and peer feedback. These workshops can cover various topics, from specific memory techniques to general cognitive exercises. Participants benefit from diverse perspectives and insights, gaining new strategies to incorporate into their routines. The collective effort in these activities reinforces the idea that learning is a shared endeavor and that we can achieve more than we ever could.

Sharing experiences and insights within a community enriches the memory improvement process. Peer-led discussions provide a platform for individuals to voice their thoughts, explore new ideas, and learn from one another. These discussions often involve overcoming specific challenges and offering practical solutions and encouragement. Personal success stories shared within the group serve as powerful inspirations. When you hear how someone else overcame a similar hurdle, it instills hope and confidence in your abilities. These stories remind us that memory improvement is achievable and that persistence pays off. They highlight the importance of community as a source of strength and motivation, a wellspring of shared wisdom and support.

Mentorship and guidance further amplify the impact of the community. Experienced individuals who have walked the path before can offer invaluable advice and motivation. Mentor-mentee relationships create a dynamic where learning is mutual, with mentors providing insights and mentees bringing fresh perspectives. This exchange fosters growth and encourages more profound understanding. Mentors can help navigate challenges, suggest tailored strategies, and offer reassurance during difficult times. Their guidance provides a roadmap, illuminating possible paths and helping to avoid common pitfalls. The presence of a mentor can make a significant difference, offering both accountability and encouragement.

Interactive Element: Community Engagement Exercise

Consider joining a local memory improvement group or an online forum. Spend time connecting with others, sharing your goals, and seeking advice on challenges you face. Take note of the insights and strategies you gain from these interactions. Reflect on how these connections influence your memory improvement journey, and consider how you might contribute to the community, sharing your own experiences and supporting others. This engagement can enrich your efforts, providing practical tips and emotional support as you enhance your memory.

9.4 TESTIMONIALS: VOICES OF THOSE WHO REMEMBER

In the past few years, I've encountered numerous individuals who have shared their heartfelt testimonials about memory improvement. These stories echo the transformative power of dedication and its profound impact on one's life. Take, for instance, John, who once struggled with remembering his daily tasks. "I used to forget appointments and birthdays," he shared. "But now, I feel more in control with consistent practice." His journey highlights the simple truth that memory enhancement is within reach for anyone willing to put in the effort. It's about finding and sticking with the proper techniques, even when going is tough.

The diversity of experiences in memory improvement is vast. Educators, for instance, often find themselves at the forefront of cognitive challenges. Emma, a high school teacher, found that her improved memory allowed her to connect more deeply with her students. "I can recall students' names and interests, which helps build rapport," she explained. Then there's Mark, a retiree, who took up memory exercises to keep his mind sharp. "I've found a new zest for life," he said, brimming with enthusiasm. These varied backgrounds remind us that memory improvement is not reserved for a select few; it spans professions and life stages, offering unique benefits to each individual's circumstances.

The emotional impact of memory improvement cannot be understated. For many, the journey results in increased confidence and self-esteem. Often, overcoming memory challenges feels like lifting a weight off one's shoulders. Linda, who once felt embarrassed by her forgetfulness, now walks with her head held high. "I feel empowered," she said, reflecting on her progress. This newfound confidence spills over into other areas of life, enhancing overall quality and satisfaction. The ability to remember details, engage fully in conversations, and participate actively in life brings immense joy and fulfillment. It's like seeing the world in full color after years of black and white.

These testimonials are potent motivators for anyone on the path to memory improvement. Real-life examples provide reassurance that change is possible. They remind us that we can make significant progress with dedication and persistence. Hearing others' stories instills hope, offering a glimpse into what could be. For those feeling discouraged or doubtful, these voices echo the sentiment that you're not alone and that success is within your grasp. The journey may be challenging, but the rewards—enhanced memory, greater confidence, and a more prosperous life—are worth the effort.

As we close this chapter, remember that memory improvement is a journey enriched by diverse experiences and shared successes. The voices captured here are a testament to what is possible with commitment and perseverance. Let these stories inspire and guide you while exploring memory enhancement techniques.

CHAPTER TEN
SUSTAINING MEMORY IMPROVEMENT FOR LIFE

Picture a thriving garden full of life. Each plant requires consistent care—watering, pruning, and nurturing—to bloom and grow. Much like this garden, your memory flourishes under the watchful eye of consistent care and routine. Establishing long-term memory habits is akin to tending this garden, ensuring that the seeds of improvement you've planted continue to grow and thrive. This chapter is about embedding these nurturing routines into your daily life, allowing you to maintain and enhance your cognitive abilities over time.

Creating consistent routines is a powerful way to support memory retention. Just as a runner benefits from a warm-up routine before a race, your brain benefits from morning rituals that include brief memory drills. Starting your day with a simple exercise, like recalling your schedule without looking at your calendar, can prime your mind for the tasks ahead. These routines prepare your brain for the day and build a foundation for long-term memory retention. Weekly review sessions serve a similar purpose. By setting aside time each week to revisit what you've learned or experienced, you reinforce those memories, making them more resistant to fading. This habit can be as simple as reflecting on the week's highlights or reviewing notes from meetings or classes, turning short-term memories into lasting knowledge.

Integrating memory exercises into daily activities might seem challenging, but with some creativity, it becomes second nature. Consider associating mundane tasks like grocery shopping with memory recall games. As you move through the store, challenge yourself to remember your list without peeking. This exercise strengthens your memory and makes a routine task more engaging. Commutes offer another opportunity for memory practice. Instead of zoning out, use this time for audio-based memory exercises. Listen to podcasts that challenge your recall or practice repeating numbers or words. These small, consistent efforts accumulate, gradually enhancing your memory without requiring significant time investment.

Maintaining motivation over time is crucial for the sustainability of these habits. One effective strategy is periodic goal reassessment. Just as a gardener observes the growth of their plants and adjusts care accordingly, regularly evaluating your memory improvement goals ensures they remain relevant and challenging. This reflection can reveal areas where you've excelled and highlight new growth opportunities. Incorporating rewards can also sustain motivation. These rewards don't need to be extravagant—simple pleasures like a favorite snack or a short walk in the park can suffice. The goal is to create positive associations with your memory practices, encouraging you to continue even when your enthusiasm wanes.

Life is dynamic, and your routines must adapt to its changes. Whether you're traveling, experiencing a busy period at work, or facing unexpected events, flexibility in your memory practices is critical. Adjust your exercises to fit your current circumstances without losing momentum. During travel, for instance, modify your routines to include portable memory games or quick recall exercises that fit your schedule. If your days become busier, adjust the frequency of your practices, ensuring they remain manageable and enjoyable. This adaptability ensures that memory improvement remains a part of your life, regardless of your changes.

Visual Element: Memory Routine Planner

Consider using a Memory Routine Planner to support the integration of these habits. This visual tool can help you organize and track your memory exercises, ensuring they fit seamlessly into your daily life. Include sections for morning rituals, weekly reviews, embedded exercises, and spaces for noting adjustments or reflections. This planner is a tangible reminder of your commitment to memory improvement, helping you stay on track.

By embedding memory improvement into your daily routines, you lay the groundwork for sustained cognitive health. These habits, though small, have a profound cumulative effect, enhancing your ability to recall and retain information over time. Just as a garden thrives with consistent care, your memory flourishes under the guidance of regular practice and mindful integration into everyday life.

10.1 FUTURE-PROOFING YOUR MEMORY: TRENDS AND INNOVATIONS

In the vast landscape of modern technology, tools are emerging that promise to revolutionize how we enhance and preserve memory. These advancements are not just futuristic concepts; they are becoming accessible and practical for everyday use. AI-driven memory coaching apps, for instance, are tailored to individual needs, offering personalized exercises and reminders. These apps learn from your interactions, adapting to your progress and providing dynamic challenges. They transform your smartphone into a memory coach, helping you stay sharp even amidst the hustle of daily life. Virtual reality (VR) environments are another groundbreaking innovation, creating immersive spaces to engage in complex memory challenges. Imagine walking through a digital landscape designed to test your recall of intricate details or to navigate a Memory Palace. These VR scenarios make learning engaging and leverage spatial memory, a powerful ally in retention.

Keeping up with cognitive science research is vital to understanding how these innovations can be optimally utilized. This field is rapidly evolving, with new findings continually reshaping our understanding of memory. Subscribing to cognitive health journals or newsletters can provide a steady stream of insights and breakthroughs. These resources often distill complex studies into practical advice, making applying the latest findings to your memory practices easier. Additionally, participating in webinars or online courses focused on brain health can offer deeper dives into specific topics. These platforms allow you to learn from experts, ask questions, and even engage in interactive sessions reinforcing your understanding. Staying informed ensures you use the most effective techniques grounded in the latest scientific research.

Innovative techniques are also gaining traction in the quest to enhance memory. Mind mapping, for example, is a method that helps process complex information. This technique involves creating a visual representation of ideas, connecting them in a way that mirrors how the brain naturally organizes information. It's particularly useful for studying or planning, as it turns abstract concepts into a structured, visual format that's easier to remember. Biofeedback devices present another intriguing development. These devices monitor physiological signals, such as heart rate and skin conductivity, providing real-time feedback on your stress levels and focus. By becoming aware of these signals, you can learn to control them, reducing stress and improving concentration. This self-regulation not only enhances memory but also contributes to overall mental well-being.

The landscape of cognitive enhancement is constantly shifting, and flexibility is critical to making the most of these changes. Being open to experimenting with different cognitive training programs lets you discover what works best. Each program may offer unique benefits, and trying various approaches can reveal unexpected strengths or preferences. Regularly updating your routines to incorporate new findings is equally essential. As science uncovers more about brain function, you can find new methods to integrate into your practice to keep it fresh and compelling. This adaptability ensures that your memory strategies remain relevant and cutting-edge, allowing you to benefit from ongoing advancements in the field.

The journey of future-proofing your memory involves embracing and integrating these innovations into your life. It's about staying curious and open to new possibilities, using technology and science to support your cognitive health. By leveraging these advancements, you can create a robust framework for memory improvement that serves you now and adapts to the challenges and opportunities of the future.

10.2 CELEBRATING YOUR MEMORY JOURNEY: MILESTONES AND ACHIEVEMENTS

In memory improvement, recognizing progress and celebrating achievements hold significant importance. It's easy to overlook the subtle victories that accumulate over time, especially when focusing on long-term goals. Yet these milestones serve as powerful reminders that progress is being made. Keeping a journal dedicated to documenting successes and breakthroughs is a tool for reflection and a testament to personal growth. Each entry can capture moments of clarity, instances where recall felt effortless, or times when a new technique just clicked. As the pages fill, they become a visual representation of your journey, offering encouragement during challenging periods when progress seems elusive. Regular reflection, perhaps at the end of each month, allows you to pause and appreciate how far you've come. This practice boosts confidence and reinforces the positive habits that enhance memory.

Sharing your success with others can amplify the joy of achievement. Whether it's family, friends, or a broader community, these sharing moments can inspire and motivate beyond your immediate circle. Hosting small gatherings to celebrate cognitive milestones creates a supportive environment where achievements are acknowledged and valued. These celebrations need not be grandiose. A simple get-together over coffee to discuss personal triumphs or hurdles can foster a sense of community and shared purpose. In today's digital age, sharing personal stories in online forums or social media can reach those on a similar path. These platforms provide a space for connection, allowing you to give and receive support. By sharing your journey, you celebrate your achievements and contribute to a culture of encouragement and growth.

Setting new challenges and goals is the natural progression after recognizing achievements. It keeps the momentum going and prevents stagnation. By continuously pushing boundaries, you open doors to further growth and discovery. Engaging in memory competitions or challenges adds an element of excitement and friendly competition. These events test your skills dynamically, offering new perspectives on your abilities. Advanced learning opportunities or certifications in fields of interest can also serve as new challenges. These pursuits enhance your knowledge and provide structured environments for applying memory techniques. As you set these new goals, consider what excites and challenges you, ensuring they align with your broader ambitions.

Reflecting on the entire journey and the lessons learned is a rewarding exercise in itself. Writing a reflective piece that captures the journey from its inception to the present can be a profound experience. This narrative allows you to trace the evolution of your memory skills, the struggles overcome, and the wisdom gained along the way. It encourages a deeper understanding of your growth, highlighting the resilience and determination that have brought you this far. Within this reflection, identify critical takeaways and future aspirations. What have you learned about yourself? What techniques have proven most effective? What areas of your life have improved as a result? These insights reinforce progress and guide future endeavors, ensuring continued growth and development.

As you continue this path of memory enhancement, remember that it's not just about the destination but also the journey. Each milestone, whether big or small, contributes to the larger picture of cognitive improvement. Celebrating these achievements fosters a positive mindset, motivating you to reach greater heights. By acknowledging progress, sharing successes, setting new challenges, and reflecting on your journey, you create a fulfilling narrative of growth and achievement; with each step, you improve your memory and enrich your life.

CONCLUSION

As we conclude this journey together, I want to reaffirm the purpose and vision that guided this book: to provide you with accessible and practical strategies for memory improvement. We've explored how simple exercises can be seamlessly woven into everyday life to enhance cognitive health. Memory is not just a static trait but a dynamic skill that can be refined and improved with dedication and effort.

In the opening chapters, we delved into understanding memory, its processes, and its challenges. Recognizing how memory works sets the stage for improvement. From there, we laid the groundwork for cognitive enhancement, exploring how your environment, nutrition, and mindfulness can bolster memory. We examined proven techniques like the Memory Palace and mnemonics, practical tools for everyday use. These chapters built a comprehensive roadmap for memory enhancement.

Chapter 9 introduced real-life success stories and testimonials that illustrate the transformative power of memory improvement. Individuals like you have faced challenges and emerged victorious, showing that enhancing memory and enriching life at any stage is possible. These stories inspire and prove that the strategies discussed in this book can lead to diverse and meaningful outcomes.

A holistic approach is essential for sustaining memory improvement. Physical health, stress management, sleep, social interaction, and lifestyle balance play pivotal roles. Together, they create a supportive environment for the brain to flourish. Embracing these elements in your routine can lead to significant cognitive enhancements.

Equally important is the role of community and support. Engaging with others who share similar goals can provide motivation and accountability. Whether through local groups or online forums, finding or creating a supportive network can amplify your efforts and foster a sense of belonging.

Now, I encourage you to take action. Implement the strategies and exercises we've discussed. Set personalized goals for your memory improvement journey and track your progress. Remember, this path requires patience and persistence. Each step is toward a sharper mind and a more fulfilling life.

Reflect on your journey so far. Celebrate your achievements, no matter how small, and identify areas for future growth. Continue exploring new techniques and adapting your routines as you progress. Memory improvement is not a destination but a continual process of learning and adaptation.

I want to express my deepest gratitude for accompanying me on this journey. It has been an honor to share this knowledge and these strategies. This book has equipped you with the tools and confidence to enhance your cognitive health and overall well-being.

As you move forward, remember that the power to improve your memory lies within you. With dedication and perseverance, you can achieve significant cognitive enhancements. Embrace the journey, celebrate your milestones, and seek new growth opportunities.

Your memory journey begins, and you have the strength and determination to succeed. Thank you for allowing me to help you on your path to a sharper, more vibrant mind.

KEEPING THE JOURNEY GOING

Now that you have the tools to enhance your memory and boost your mental clarity, it's time to share your journey with others. The insights you've gained can inspire someone else to take their first steps toward better cognitive health.

By leaving your honest review of **Memory Fitness Revolution** on Amazon, you're helping others discover the guidance they need. Your feedback could point someone toward the exercises, strategies, and tips that made a difference for you, creating a ripple effect of positive change.

Your voice matters. Together, we can help more people unlock their potential and improve their lives.

Thank you for your support. Building sharper minds and stronger memories is a journey we can take together, and by sharing your experience, you're making that possible.

>>> Click here to leave your review on Amazon.

REFERENCES

Hippocampus: What It Is, Function, Location & Damage https://my.clevelandclinic.org/health/body/hippocampus#:

How to Rewire Your Brain: 6 Neuroplasticity Exercises https://www.healthline.com/health/rewiring-your-brain

Effects of stress hormones on the brain and cognition https://pmc.ncbi.nlm.nih.gov/articles/PMC5619133/

Memory: Myth Versus Truth https://www.hopkinsmedicine.org/health/wellness-and-prevention/memory-myth-versus-truth

The benefit of inhalation aromatherapy as a complementary ... https://www.sciencedirect.com/science/article/pii/S1744388123000312

Effects of Omega-3 Polyunsaturated Fatty Acids on Brain ... https://pubmed.ncbi.nlm.nih.gov/36381743/

Mindfulness exercises https://www.mayoclinic.org/healthy-lifestyle/consumer-health/in-depth/mindfulness-exercises/art-20046356

Neuroplasticity exercises: 5 tips to try https://www.medicalnewstoday.com/articles/neuroplasticity-exercises

Method of loci https://en.wikipedia.org/wiki/Method_of_loci

Mnemonic Devices: Types, Examples, and Benefits https://psychcentral.com/lib/memory-and-mnemonic-devices

How Chunking Pieces of Information Can Improve Memory https://www.verywellmind.com/chunking-how-can-this-technique-improve-your-memory-2794969

Spaced repetition (article) | Learn to Learn | Khan Academy https://www.khanacademy.org/science/learn-to-learn/x141050afa14cfed3:learn-to-learn/x141050afa14cfed3:spaced-repetition/a/l2l-spaced-repetition#:

10 Simple Morning Habits to Improve Your Brain and Day https://thebestbrainpossible.com/brain-health-healthy-performance-prevention/

14 Neurobic Exercises For Brain Exercise And Better Memory https://www.magneticmemorymethod.com/neurobics/

Expressive writing can increase working memory capacity https://pubmed.ncbi.nlm.nih.gov/11561925/

Enhancing Cognitive Abilities: The Impact of Memory ... https://junilearning.com/blog/guide/enhancing-cognitive-abilities/

13 Brain Exercises to Help Keep You Mentally Sharp https://www.healthline.com/health/mental-health/brain-exercises

REFERENCES

Science-Backed Memory Tips and Recall Techniques https://www.usa.edu/blog/science-backed-memory-tips/

Neuroscientists Unlock the Secrets of Memory Champions https://www.smithsonianmag.com/science-nature/why-you-can-train-your-brain-memory-champion-still-forget-your-car-keys-180962496/

Can Brain Games Improve Cognitive Ability? | St. Luke's Health https://www.stlukeshealth.org/resources/can-brain-games-improve-cognitive-ability

These training apps are a workout for your brain - Deseret News https://www.deseret.com/23855667/brain-training-apps/.

Effects of Virtual Reality-Based Cognitive Training in the ... https://pmc.ncbi.nlm.nih.gov/articles/PMC8328838/

Gamification of Cognitive Assessment and Cognitive Training https://pmc.ncbi.nlm.nih.gov/articles/PMC4967181/

Digital technologies for the assessment of cognition https://www.ncbi.nlm.nih.gov/pmc/articles/PMC10270380/

Medical myths about aging: Is deterioration inevitable? https://www.medicalnewstoday.com/articles/medical-myths-all-about-aging

Improve your working memory with 60 quick exercises: https://eatspeakthink.com/improve-working-memory-60-exercises/

Mechanisms of motivation–cognition interaction https://pmc.ncbi.nlm.nih.gov/articles/PMC4986920/

Memory Clinic: Living with Memory Disorders https://gwdocs.com/specialties/memory-clinic/living-with-memory-disorders

How Exercise Protects Your Brain's Health https://health.clevelandclinic.org/exercise-and-brain-health

Stress effects on the hippocampus: a critical review - PMC https://pmc.ncbi.nlm.nih.gov/articles/PMC4561403/

Sleep stages and memory https://www.health.harvard.edu/healthbeat/sleep-stages-and-memory

Associations between social connections and cognition https://www.ncbi.nlm.nih.gov/pmc/articles/PMC9750173/

The Father of Modern Memory Improvement Harry Lorayne https://superhumanacademy.com/podcast/the-father-of-modern-memory-improvement-harry-lorayne-60-years-of-mnemonics/

An effortless way to improve your memory https://www.bbc.com/future/article/20180208-an-effortless-way-to-strengthen-your-memory

Social Support and Cognition: A Systematic Review https://www.frontiersin.org/journals/psychology/articles/10.3389/fpsyg.2021.637060/full

How I Used The Memory Palace To Write My Exam Essays ... https://benjaminmcevoy.com/how-i-used-the-memory-palace-to-write-my-exam-essays-at-oxford/

How Establishing a Routine Can Improve Memory for ... https://www.irisseniorliving.com/senior-living/ok/oklahoma-city/n-may-ave/blog/how-establishing-a-routine-can-improve-memory-for-individuals-with-memory-loss

Can neurotechnology revolutionize cognitive enhancement? https://journals.plos.org/plosbiology/article?id=10.1371/journal.pbio.3002831

Mind Mastery: 15 Proven Memory Techniques https://learnlever.com/master-15-proven-memory-techniques-october-2023/

Importance of Cognitive Milestones in Early Childhood https://growingwithnemit.com/importance-cognitive-milestones/

www.ingramcontent.com/pod-product-compliance
Lightning Source LLC
Chambersburg PA
CBHW070635030426
42337CB00020B/4024